CONTENTS

BREAKFAST RECIPES

1. Tortilla De Patatas With Spinach

Servings: 4
Cooking Time: 25 Minutes
Ingredients:
- 3 cups potato cubes, boiled
- 2 cups spinach, chopped
- 5 eggs, lightly beaten
- ¼ cup heavy cream
- 1 cup mozzarella cheese, grated
- ½ cup fresh parsley, chopped
- Salt and black pepper to taste

Directions:
1. Preheat Breville on Bake function to 390 F. Place the potatoes in a greased baking dish. In a bowl, whisk eggs, heavy cream, spinach, mozzarella cheese, parsley, salt, and pepper and pour over the potatoes. Press Start. Cook for 16 minutes until nice and golden. Serve warm.

2. Bulgogi Burgers

Servings: 4
Cooking Time: 10 Minutes
Ingredients:
- Burgers:
- 1 pound (454 g) 85% lean ground beef
- 2 tablespoons gochujang
- ¼ cup chopped scallions
- 2 teaspoons minced garlic
- 2 teaspoons minced fresh ginger
- 1 tablespoon soy sauce
- 1 tablespoon toasted sesame oil
- 2 teaspoons sugar
- ½ teaspoon kosher salt
- 4 hamburger buns
- Cooking spray
- Korean Mayo:
- 1 tablespoon gochujang
- ¼ cup mayonnaise
- 2 teaspoons sesame seeds
- ¼ cup chopped scallions
- 1 tablespoon toasted sesame oil

Directions:
1. Combine the ingredients for the burgers, except for the buns, in a large bowl. Stir to mix well, then wrap the bowl in plastic and refrigerate to marinate for at least an hour.
2. Spritz the air fryer basket with cooking spray.
3. Divide the meat mixture into four portions and form into four balls. Bash the balls into patties.
4. Arrange the patties in the pan and spritz with cooking spray.
5. Put the air fryer basket on the baking pan and slide into Rack Position 2, select Air Fry, set temperature to 350ºF (180ºC) and set time to 10 minutes.
6. Flip the patties halfway through the cooking time.
7. Meanwhile, combine the ingredients for the Korean mayo in a small bowl. Stir to mix well.
8. When cooking is complete, the patties should be golden brown.
9. Remove the patties from the oven and assemble with the buns, then spread the Korean mayo over the patties to make the burgers. Serve immediately.

3. Poppy Seed Muffins

Servings: 12
Cooking Time: 20 Minutes
Ingredients:
- 3 tbsp poppy seeds
- 1 tsp vanilla
- 8 tbsp maple syrup
- 2 tbsp lemon zest
- 6 tbsp lemon juice
- 4/5 cup almond milk
- 1/4 cup butter, melted
- 1/4 tsp baking soda
- 2 tsp baking powder
- 1 1/4 cups flour
- 1 1/4 cups almond flour
- Pinch of salt

Directions:
1. Fit the oven with the rack in position
2. Line 12-cups muffin tin with cupcake liners and set aside.
3. In a large bowl, mix together melted butter, milk, lemon zest, vanilla, lemon juice, poppy seeds, maple syrup, and almond flour.
4. Add flour, baking soda, and baking powder. Stir until well combined.
5. Pour batter into the prepared muffin tin.
6. Set to bake at 350 F for 25 minutes, after 5 minutes, place the muffin tin in the oven.
7. Serve and enjoy.

Nutrition Info: Calories 239 Fat 14.4 g Carbohydrates 23.6 g Sugar 9.1 g Protein 4.7 g Cholesterol 10 mg

4. Corn & Chorizo Frittata

Servings: 2
Cooking Time: 20 Minutes
Ingredients:
- 4 eggs

- 1 large potato, boiled and cubed
- ½ cup frozen corn
- ½ cup feta cheese, crumbled
- 1 tbsp fresh parsley, chopped
- ½ chorizo, sliced
- 1 tbsp olive oil
- Salt and black pepper to taste

Directions:

1. Preheat on Air Fry function to 375 F. Heat the olive oil in a skillet over medium heat and cook the chorizo cook for 3 minutes. Beat the eggs with salt and pepper in a bowl. Stir in chorizo and the remaining ingredients. Pour the mixture into the baking pan of oven and cook for 10-15 minutes on Bake function. Serve sliced.

5. Nutmeg Potato Gratin

Servings: 5
Cooking Time: 45 Minutes
Ingredients:

- 5 large potatoes
- ½ cup sour cream
- ½ cup grated cheese
- ½ cup milk
- ½ tsp nutmeg
- Salt and black pepper to taste

Directions:

1. Preheat on Bake function to 375 F, peel and slice the potatoes. In a bowl, combine the sour cream, milk, pepper, salt, and nutmeg. Add in the potato slices and stir to coat them well.
2. Transfer the mixture to an ovenproof casserole. Cook for 15 minutes on Bake function, then sprinkle the cheese on top and cook for 10 minutes. Allow to sit for 10 minutes before serving.

6. Sweet Pineapple Oatmeal

Servings: 6
Cooking Time: 45 Minutes
Ingredients:

- 2 cups old-fashioned oats
- 1/2 cup coconut flakes
- 1 cup pineapple, crushed
- 2 eggs, lightly beaten
- 1/3 cup yogurt
- 1/3 cup butter, melted
- 1/2 tsp baking powder
- 1/3 cup brown sugar
- 1/2 tsp vanilla
- 2/3 cup milk
- 1/2 tsp salt

Directions:

1. Fit the oven with the rack in position

2. In a mixing bowl, mix together oats, baking powder, brown sugar, and salt.
3. In a separate bowl, beat eggs with vanilla, milk, yogurt, and butter.
4. Add egg mixture into the oat mixture and stir to combine.
5. Add coconut and pineapple and stir to combine.
6. Pour oat mixture into the greased 8-inch baking dish.
7. Set to bake at 350 F for 50 minutes, after 5 minutes, place the baking dish in the oven.
8. Serve and enjoy.

Nutrition Info: Calories 304 Fat 16.4 g Carbohydrates 33.2 g Sugar 13.6 g Protein 7.5 g Cholesterol 85 mg

7. Air Fried Crispy Spring Rolls

Servings: 4
Cooking Time: 18 Minutes
Ingredients:

- 4 spring roll wrappers
- ½ cup cooked vermicelli noodles
- 1 teaspoon sesame oil
- 1 tablespoon freshly minced ginger
- 1 tablespoon soy sauce
- 1 clove garlic, minced
- ½ red bell pepper, deseeded and chopped
- ½ cup chopped carrot
- ½ cup chopped mushrooms
- ¼ cup chopped scallions
- Cooking spray

Directions:

1. Spritz the air fryer basket with cooking spray and set aside.
2. Heat the sesame oil in a saucepan on medium heat. Sauté the ginger and garlic in the sesame oil for 1 minute, or until fragrant. Add soy sauce, red bell pepper, carrot, mushrooms and scallions. Sauté for 5 minutes or until the vegetables become tender. Mix in vermicelli noodles. Turn off the heat and remove them from the saucepan. Allow to cool for 10 minutes.
3. Lay out one spring roll wrapper with a corner pointed toward you. Scoop the noodle mixture on spring roll wrapper and fold corner up over the mixture. Fold left and right corners toward the center and continue to roll to make firmly sealed rolls.
4. Arrange the spring rolls in the pan and spritz with cooking spray.
5. Put the air fryer basket on the baking pan and slide into Rack Position 2, select Air Fry, set temperature to 340ºF (171ºC) and set time to 12 minutes.
6. Flip the spring rolls halfway through the cooking time.

7. When done, the spring rolls will be golden brown and crispy.
8. Serve warm.

8. Chives Salmon And Shrimp Bowls

Servings: 4
Cooking Time: 12 Minutes
Ingredients:
- 1 pound shrimp, peeled and deveined
- ½ pound salmon fillets, boneless and cubed
- 2 spring onions, chopped
- 2 teaspoons olive oil
- 1 cup baby kale
- Salt and black pepper to the taste
- 1 tablespoon chives, chopped
Directions:
1. Preheat the air fryer with the oil at 330 degrees F, add the shrimp, salmon and the other ingredients, toss gently and cook for 12 minutes.
2. Divide everything into bowls and serve.
Nutrition Info: calories 244, fat 11, fiber 4, carbs 5, protein 7

9. Asparagus And Cheese Strata

Servings: 4
Cooking Time: 17 Minutes
Ingredients:
- 6 asparagus spears, cut into 2-inch pieces
- 1 tablespoon water
- 2 slices whole-wheat bread, cut into ½-inch cubes
- 4 eggs
- 3 tablespoons whole milk
- 2 tablespoons chopped flat-leaf parsley
- ½ cup grated Havarti or Swiss cheese
- Pinch salt
- Freshly ground black pepper, to taste
- Cooking spray
Directions:
1. Add the asparagus spears and 1 tablespoon of water in the baking pan.
2. Slide the baking pan into Rack Position 1, select Convection Bake, set temperature to 330ºF (166ºC) and set time to 4 minutes.
3. When cooking is complete, the asparagus spears will be crisp-tender.
4. Remove the asparagus from the pan and drain on paper towels.
5. Spritz the pan with cooking spray. Place the bread and asparagus in the pan.
6. Whisk together the eggs and milk in a medium mixing bowl until creamy. Fold in the parsley, cheese,

salt, and pepper and stir to combine. Pour this mixture into the baking pan.
7. Select Bake and set time to 13 minutes. Put the pan back to the oven. When done, the eggs will be set and the top will be lightly browned.
8. Let cool for 5 minutes before slicing and serving.

10. Cauliflower And Cod Mix

Servings: 4
Cooking Time: 20 Minutes
Ingredients:
- 2 cups cauliflower florets
- 1-pound cod fillets, boneless and cubed
- 1 cup baby spinach
- 1 cup baby arugula
- 1 tablespoon olive oil
- 1 teaspoon sweet paprika
- 1 teaspoon rosemary, dried
- A pinch of salt and black pepper
Directions:
1. Heat up your air fryer with the oil at 340 degrees F, add the cauliflower, cod and the other ingredients, toss gently and cook for 20 minutes.
2. Divide the mix into bowls and serve for breakfast.
Nutrition Info: calories 240, fat 9, fiber 2, carbs 4, protein 8

11. Cheesy Baked-egg Toast

Servings: 4
Cooking Time: 10 Minutes
Ingredients:
- 4 slices wheat bread
- 4 eggs
- 1 cup shredded cheese
- 2 tablespoons softened butter
Directions:
1. Start by preheating toaster oven to 350°F.
2. Place bread on a greased baking sheet.
3. Use a teaspoon to push a square into the bread creating a little bed for the egg.
4. Sprinkle salt and pepper over the bread.
5. Break one egg into each square. Spread butter over each edge of the bread.
6. Sprinkle 1/4 cup cheese over buttered area.
7. Bake for 10 minutes or until the eggs are solid and the cheese is golden brown.
Nutrition Info: Calories: 297, Sodium: 410 mg, Dietary Fiber: 1.9 g, Total Fat: 20.4 g, Total Carbs: 12.3 g, Protein: 16.3 g.

12. Chicken Breakfast Sausages

Servings: 8 Patties
Cooking Time: 10 Minutes
Ingredients:
- 1 Granny Smith apple, peeled and finely chopped
- 2 tablespoons apple juice
- 2 garlic cloves, minced
- 1 egg white
- $1/_3$ cup minced onion
- 3 tablespoons ground almonds
- ⅛ teaspoon freshly ground black pepper
- 1 pound (454 g) ground chicken breast

Directions:
1. Combine all the ingredients except the chicken in a medium mixing bowl and stir well.
2. Add the chicken breast to the apple mixture and mix with your hands until well incorporated.
3. Divide the mixture into 8 equal portions and shape into patties. Arrange the patties in the air fryer basket.
4. Put the air fryer basket on the baking pan and slide into Rack Position 2, select Air Fry, set temperature to 330ºF (166ºC) and set time to 10 minutes.
5. When done, a meat thermometer inserted in the center of the chicken should reach at least 165ºF (74ºC).
6. Remove from the oven to a plate. Let the chicken cool for 5 minutes and serve warm.

13. Apricot & Almond Scones

Servings: 4
Cooking Time: 30 Minutes
Ingredients:
- 2 cups flour
- ⅓ cup sugar
- 2 tsp baking powder
- ½ cup sliced almonds
- ¾ cup dried apricots, chopped
- ¼ cup cold butter, cut into cubes
- ½ cup milk
- 1 egg
- 1 tsp vanilla extract

Directions:
1. reheat Breville on AirFry function to 370 F. Line a baking dish with parchment paper. Mix together flour, sugar, baking powder, almonds, and apricots. Rub the butter into the dry ingredients with hands to form a sandy, crumbly texture. Whisk together egg, milk, and vanilla extract.
2. Pour into the dry ingredients and stir to combine. Sprinkle a working board with flour, lay the dough onto the board and give it a few kneads. Shape into a rectangle and cut into 8 squares. Arrange the

squares on the baking dish and press Start. Bake for 25 minutes. Serve chilled.

14. Nutritious Cinnamon Oat Muffins

Servings: 12
Cooking Time: 30 Minutes
Ingredients:
- 2 cups oat flour
- 1/3 cup coconut oil, melted
- 1/2 cup maple syrup
- 1 cup applesauce
- 1 tsp cinnamon
- 2 tsp baking powder
- 1 tsp vanilla
- 1/4 tsp salt

Directions:
1. Fit the oven with the rack in position
2. Line 12-cups muffin tin with cupcake liners and set aside.
3. In a bowl, add applesauce, cinnamon, vanilla, oil, maple syrup, and salt and stir to combine.
4. Add baking powder and oat flour and stir well.
5. Pour batter into the prepared muffin tin.
6. Set to bake at 350 F for 35 minutes, after 5 minutes, place the muffin tin in the oven.
7. Serve and enjoy.
Nutrition Info: Calories 158 Fat 7.1 g Carbohydrates 22.2 g Sugar 9.9 g Protein 2 g Cholesterol 0 mg

15. Egg Ham Casserole

Servings: 2
Cooking Time: 20 Minutes
Ingredients:
- 5 eggs, lightly beaten
- 1 slice bread, cut into pieces
- 1/3 cup ham, diced
- 1 tbsp pimento, diced
- 1/2 cup cheddar cheese, shredded
- 1/3 cup heavy cream
- 2 green onion, chopped
- 1/4 tsp black pepper
- 1/4 tsp salt

Directions:
1. Fit the oven with the rack in position
2. Add bread pieces to the bottom of the greased casserole dish.
3. In a bowl, whisk eggs with heavy cream, pimento, green onion, pepper, and salt.
4. Pour egg mixture over bread.
5. Sprinkle ham and cheese over egg mixture.
6. Set to bake at 350 F for 25 minutes. After 5 minutes place the casserole dish in the preheated oven.

7. Serve and enjoy.

Nutrition Info: Calories 413 Fat 30 g Carbohydrates 10.7 g Sugar 4.6 g Protein 26.3 g Cholesterol 479 mg

16. Amazing Apple & Brie Sandwich

Servings: 1
Cooking Time: 10 Minutes
Ingredients:

- 2 bread slices
- ½ apple, thinly sliced
- 2 tsp butter
- 2 oz brie cheese, thinly sliced

Directions:
1. Spread butter on the outside of the bread slices. Arrange apple slices on the inside of one bread slice. Place brie slices on top of the apple. Top with the other slice of bread. Press Start on the Breville oven and cook for 5 minutes at 350 F on Bake function. Cut diagonally and serve.

17. Air Fried Philly Cheesesteaks

Servings: 2
Cooking Time: 20 Minutes
Ingredients:

- 12 ounces (340 g) boneless rib-eye steak, sliced thinly
- ½ teaspoon Worcestershire sauce
- ½ teaspoon soy sauce
- Kosher salt and ground black pepper, to taste
- ½ green bell pepper, stemmed, deseeded, and thinly sliced
- ½ small onion, halved and thinly sliced
- 1 tablespoon vegetable oil
- 2 soft hoagie rolls, split three-fourths of the way through
- 1 tablespoon butter, softened
- 2 slices provolone cheese, halved

Directions:
1. Combine the steak, Worcestershire sauce, soy sauce, salt, and ground black pepper in a large bowl. Toss to coat well. Set aside.
2. Combine the bell pepper, onion, salt, ground black pepper, and vegetable oil in a separate bowl. Toss to coat the vegetables well.
3. Place the steak and vegetables in the air fryer basket.
4. Put the air fryer basket on the baking pan and slide into Rack Position 2, select Air Fry, set temperature to 400ºF (205ºC) and set time to 15 minutes.
5. When cooked, the steak will be browned and vegetables will be tender. Transfer them onto a plate. Set aside.

6. Brush the hoagie rolls with butter and place in the basket.
7. Select Toast and set time to 3 minutes. Return to the oven. When done, the rolls should be lightly browned.
8. Transfer the rolls to a clean work surface and divide the steak and vegetable mix between the rolls. Spread with cheese. Transfer the stuffed rolls to the basket.
9. Select Air Fry and set time to 2 minutes. Return to the oven. When done, the cheese should be melted.
10. Serve immediately.

18. Healthy Oatmeal Bars

Servings: 18
Cooking Time: 20 Minutes
Ingredients:

- 2 cups oatmeal
- 1/2 tsp allspice
- 1 tsp baking soda
- 1 tbsp maple syrup
- 1 cup butter
- 1 cup of sugar
- 1 cup flour

Directions:
1. Fit the oven with the rack in position
2. Add butter and maple syrup into a bowl and microwave until butter is melted. Stir well.
3. In a mixing bowl, mix oatmeal, sugar, flour, allspice, and baking soda.
4. Add melted butter and maple syrup mixture and mix until well combined.
5. Pour mixture into the parchment-lined 9*12-inch baking dish. Spread well.
6. Set to bake at 350 F for 25 minutes, after 5 minutes, place the baking dish in the oven.
7. Slice and serve.

Nutrition Info: Calories 195 Fat 10.9 g Carbohydrates 23.4 g Sugar 11.9 g Protein 2 g Cholesterol 27 mg

19. Veggies Breakfast Salad

Servings: 4
Cooking Time: 15 Minutes
Ingredients:

- 2 tablespoons olive oil
- 1 cup cherry tomatoes, halved
- 1 zucchini, cubed
- 1 eggplant, cubed
- 1 red onion, chopped
- 1 fennel bulb, shredded
- 1 cup cheddar, shredded
- 2 tablespoons chives, chopped

- Salt and black pepper to the taste
- 8 eggs, whisked

Directions:
1. Add the oil to your air fryer, heat it up at 350 degrees F, add the onion and fennel and cook for 2 minutes.
2. Add the tomatoes and the other ingredients except the cheese and toss.
3. Sprinkle the cheese on top, cook the mix for 13 minutes more, divide into bowls and serve for breakfast.

Nutrition Info: calories 221, fat 8, fiber 3, carbs 4, protein 8

20. Mini Cinnamon Rolls

Servings: 18 Rolls
Cooking Time: 25 Minutes
Ingredients:
- $^1/_3$ cup light brown sugar
- 2 teaspoons cinnamon
- 1 (9-by-9-inch) frozen puff pastry sheet, thawed
- All-purpose flour, for dusting
- 6 teaspoons unsalted butter, melted, divided

Directions:
1. In a small bowl, stir together the brown sugar and cinnamon.
2. On a clean work surface, lightly dust with the flour and lay the puff pastry sheet. Using a rolling pin, press the folds together and roll the dough out in one direction so that it measures about 9 by 11 inches. Cut it in half to form two squat rectangles of about 5½ by 9 inches.
3. Brush 2 teaspoons of the butter over each pastry half. Sprinkle with 2 tablespoons of the cinnamon sugar. Pat it down lightly with the palm of your hand to help it adhere to the butter.
4. Starting with the 9-inch side of one rectangle. Using your hands, carefully roll the dough into a cylinder. Repeat with the other rectangle. To make slicing easier, refrigerate the rolls for 10 to 20 minutes.
5. Using a sharp knife, slice each roll into nine 1-inch pieces. Transfer the rolls to the center of the baking pan. They should be very close to each other, but not quite touching. Drizzle the remaining 2 teaspoons of the butter over the rolls and sprinkle with the remaining cinnamon sugar.
6. Slide the baking pan into Rack Position 1, select Convection Bake, set temperature to 350ºF (180ºC) and set time to 25 minutes.
7. When cooking is complete, remove the pan and check the rolls. They should be puffed up and golden brown.
8. Let the rolls rest for 5 minutes and transfer them to a wire rack to cool completely. Serve.

21. Cheesy Potato Taquitos

Servings: 12 Taquitos
Cooking Time: 6 Minutes
Ingredients:
- 2 cups mashed potatoes
- ½ cup shredded Mexican cheese
- 12 corn tortillas
- Cooking spray

Directions:
1. Line the baking pan with parchment paper.
2. In a bowl, combine the potatoes and cheese until well mixed. Microwave the tortillas on high heat for 30 seconds, or until softened. Add some water to another bowl and set alongside.
3. On a clean work surface, lay the tortillas. Scoop 3 tablespoons of the potato mixture in the center of each tortilla. Roll up tightly and secure with toothpicks if necessary.
4. Arrange the filled tortillas, seam side down, in the prepared baking pan. Spritz the tortillas with cooking spray.
5. Put the air fryer basket on the baking pan and slide into Rack Position 2, select Air Fry, set temperature to 400ºF (205ºC) and set time to 6 minutes.
6. Flip the tortillas halfway through the cooking time.
7. When cooked, the tortillas should be crispy and golden brown.
8. Serve hot.

22. Savory Cheddar & Cauliflower Tater Tots

Servings: 4
Cooking Time: 35 Minutes
Ingredients:
- 2 lb cauliflower florets, steamed
- 5 oz cheddar cheese, shredded
- 1 onion, diced
- 1 cup breadcrumbs
- 1 egg, beaten
- 1 tsp fresh parsley, chopped
- 1 tsp fresh oregano, chopped
- 1 tsp fresh chives, chopped
- 1 tsp garlic powder
- Salt and black pepper to taste

Directions:
1. Mash the cauliflower and place it in a large bowl. Add in the onion, parsley, oregano, chives, garlic powder, salt, pepper, and cheddar cheese. Mix with your hands until thoroughly combined and form 12 balls out of the mixture.

2. Line a baking sheet with parchment paper. Dip half of the tater tots into the egg and then coat with breadcrumbs. Arrange them on the AirFryer Basket and spray with cooking spray.
3. Fit in the baking sheet and cook in the fryer oven at 390 minutes for 10-12 minutes on Air Fry function. Serve.

23. Vanilla & Cinnamon Toast Toppet

Servings: 6
Cooking Time: 10 Minutes
Ingredients:
- 12 slices bread
- ½ cup sugar
- 1 ½ tsp cinnamon
- 1 stick of butter, softened
- 1 tsp vanilla extract

Directions:
1. Preheat on Toast function to 360 F. Combine all ingredients, except the bread, in a bowl. Spread the buttery cinnamon mixture onto the bread slices. Place the bread slices in the toaster oven. Cook for 8 minutes. Serve.

24. Cinnamon Streusel Bread

Servings: 8
Cooking Time: 30 Minutes
Ingredients:
- 1 cup warm water
- 1 envelope yeast, quick rising
- 1/3 cup + 6 tsp milk, divided
- 1 egg
- 3 tbsp. sugar
- 3 ½ cups flour, divided
- 1 tbsp. + 2 tsp olive oil
- 1 tsp salt
- 2 tbsp. cinnamon
- ½ cup brown sugar
- 2 tbsp. butter, cold & cut in cubes
- 1 cup powdered sugar

Directions:
1. In a large bowl, add water and sprinkle yeast over top, stir to dissolve.
2. Stir in 1/3 cup milk, egg, and sugar until combined.
3. Add 2 cups flour and stir in until batter gets thick. With a wooden spoon, or mixer with dough hook attached, beat 100 strokes.
4. Fold in oil and salt. Then stir in 1 ¼ cups flour until dough begins to come together.
5. Mix in cinnamon and transfer dough to a lightly floured work surface. Knead for 5 minutes then form into a ball.

6. Use remaining oil to grease a clean bowl and add dough. Cover and let rise 30 minutes.
7. Spray a 9-inch loaf pan with cooking spray.
8. After 30 minutes, punch dough down and divide into 8 equal pieces.
9. Place brown sugar in a shallow bowl and roll dough pieces in it, forming it into balls. Place in prepared pan and sprinkle remaining brown sugar over top.
10. In a small bowl, combine butter and ¼ cup flour until mixture resembles coarse crumbs. Sprinkle over top of bread.
11. Place rack in position 1 of the oven. Set to convection bake on 325°F and set timer for 35 minutes. After 5 minutes, add pan to the rack and bake 30 minutes or until golden brown.
12. Let cool in pan 10 minutes, then invert onto wire rack.
13. In a small bowl, whisk together powdered sugar and milk until smooth. Drizzle over warm bread and serve.
Nutrition Info: Calories 328, Total Fat 6g, Saturated Fat 2g, Total Carbs 60g, Net Carbs 58g, Protein 6g, Sugar 25g, Fiber 2g, Sodium 266mg, Potassium 94mg, Phosphorus 71mg

25. Soft Banana Oat Muffins

Servings: 12
Cooking Time: 20 Minutes
Ingredients:
- 1 egg
- 1 cup banana, mashed
- 1 tsp vanilla
- 1/3 cup applesauce
- 3/4 cup milk
- 1/4 tsp nutmeg
- 1/2 tsp cinnamon
- 1 tsp baking soda
- 2 tsp baking powder
- 1/4 cup brown sugar
- 1/4 cup white sugar
- 1 cup old fashioned oats
- 1 1/2 cups whole wheat flour
- 1/2 tsp salt

Directions:
1. Fit the oven with the rack in position
2. Line a 12-cup muffin tray with cupcake liners and set aside.
3. In a mixing bowl, mix flour, nutmeg, cinnamon, baking soda, baking powder, sugar, oats, flour, and salt.
4. In a separate bowl, whisk eggs with milk, vanilla, and applesauce. Add mashed banana and stir to combine.

5. Add flour mixture into the egg mixture and mix until just combined.
6. Pour mixture into the prepared muffin tray.
7. Set to bake at 400 F for 25 minutes. After 5 minutes place the muffin tray in the preheated oven.
8. Serve and enjoy.
Nutrition Info: Calories 165 Fat 1.7 g Carbohydrates 33 g Sugar 10.5 g Protein 4.4 g Cholesterol 15 mg

26. Healthy Squash

Servings: 4
Cooking Time: 25 Minutes
Ingredients:
- 2 lbs yellow squash, cut into half-moons
- 1 tsp Italian seasoning
- ¼ tsp pepper
- 1 tbsp olive oil
- ¼ tsp salt

Directions:
1. Add all ingredients into the large bowl and toss well.
2. Preheat the air fryer to 400 F.
3. Add squash mixture into the air fryer basket and cook for 10 minutes.
4. Shake basket and cook for another 10 minutes.
5. Shake once again and cook for 5 minutes more.
Nutrition Info: Calories 70, Fat 4 g, Carbohydrates 7 g, Sugar 4 g, Protein 2 g, Cholesterol 1 mg

27. Smart Oven Jalapeño Popper Grilled Cheese Recipe

Ingredients:
- 1 medium Jalapeño
- 2 slices Whole Grain Bread
- 2 teaspoons Mayonnaise
- 1/2-ounce Shredded Mild Cheddar Cheese, (about 2 tablespoons)
- 2 teaspoons Honey
- 1-ounce Cream Cheese, softened
- 1 tablespoon Sliced Green Onions
- dash of Garlic Powder
- 1-ounce Shredded Monterey Jack Cheese, (about 1/4 cup)
- 1/4 cup Corn Flakes Cereal

Directions:
1. Cut jalapeño into 1/4-inch slices. If you want your Classic Sandwich less spicy, use a paring knife to remove the seeds and veins.
2. Adjust cooking rack to the top placement and select the BROIL setting. Place jalapeño slices on a baking sheet, and broil until they have softened and are just starting to brown, about 2 to 4 minutes. Remove pan and set aside.

3. Adjust the cooking rack to the bottom position. Place an empty sheet pan inside of the toaster oven, and preheat to 400°F on the BAKE setting.
4. Spread one side of each slice of bread with mayonnaise. Place the bread mayo-side-down on a cutting board.
5. In a small bowl, combine the cream cheese, green onion, and garlic powder. Spread each slice of bread with the mixture. Arrange jalapeño slices in an even layer on one slice and distribute the cheese evenly over both pieces of bread.
6. Carefully remove the pan and add the bread, mayo-side-down, to the pan. Return to the oven and bake until the bread is toasted and the cheese is melted and bubbly, about 6 to 7 minutes.
7. Finishing Touches
8. Drizzle the honey over the jalapeño and sprinkle with corn flakes. Immediately top with the remaining cheesy bread slice.

28. Creamy Parmesan & Ham Shirred Eggs

Servings: 2
Cooking Time: 20 Minutes
Ingredients:
- 2 tsp butter
- 4 eggs, divided
- 2 tbsp heavy cream
- 4 slices of ham
- 3 tbsp Parmesan cheese, shredded
- ¼ tsp paprika
- ¾ tsp salt
- ¼ tsp pepper
- 2 tsp chopped chives

Directions:
1. Preheat on Bake function to 320 F. Grease a pie pan with the butter. Arrange the ham slices on the bottom of the pan to cover it completely. Whisk one egg along with the heavy cream, salt, and pepper in a bowl.
2. Pour the mixture over the ham slices. Crack the other eggs over the ham. Sprinkle with Parmesan cheese. Cook for 14 minutes. Season with paprika, garnish with chives, and serve.

29. Perfect Potato Casserole

Servings: 6
Cooking Time: 35 Minutes
Ingredients:
- 32 oz shredded potatoes
- 1/4 cup milk
- 1/4 cup butter, melted
- 1 cup cheddar cheese, shredded

- 10.5 oz cheddar cheese soup
- 2/3 cup sour cream
- 1/2 tsp onion powder
- 1/2 tsp garlic powder

Directions:
1. Fit the oven with the rack in position
2. Spray 9*13-inch baking pan with cooking spray and set aside.
3. Add all ingredients into the greased baking pan and mix well.
4. Set to bake at 350 F for 40 minutes. After 5 minutes place the baking pan in the preheated oven.
5. Serve and enjoy.

Nutrition Info: Calories 341 Fat 21.7 g Carbohydrates 28 g Sugar 2.5 g Protein 9.6 g Cholesterol 58 mg

30. Egg And Avocado Burrito

Servings: 4
Cooking Time: 4 Minutes
Ingredients:
- 4 low-sodium whole-wheat flour tortillas
- Filling:
- 1 hard-boiled egg, chopped
- 2 hard-boiled egg whites, chopped
- 1 ripe avocado, peeled, pitted, and chopped
- 1 red bell pepper, chopped
- 1 (1.2-ounce / 34-g) slice low-sodium, low-fat American cheese, torn into pieces
- 3 tablespoons low-sodium salsa, plus additional for serving (optional)
- Special Equipment:
- 4 toothpicks (optional), soaked in water for at least 30 minutes

Directions:
1. Make the filling: Combine the egg, egg whites, avocado, red bell pepper, cheese, and salsa in a medium bowl and stir until blended.
2. Assemble the burritos: Arrange the tortillas on a clean work surface and place ¼ of the prepared filling in the middle of each tortilla, leaving about 1½-inch on each end unfilled. Fold in the opposite sides of each tortilla and roll up. Secure with toothpicks through the center, if needed.
3. Transfer the burritos to the air fryer basket.
4. Put the air fryer basket on the baking pan and slide into Rack Position 2, select Air Fry, set temperature to 390ºF (199ºC) and set time to 4 minutes.
5. When cooking is complete, the burritos should be crisp and golden brown.
6. Allow to cool for 5 minutes and serve with salsa, if desired.

31. Baked Avocado With Eggs

Servings: 2
Cooking Time: 9 Minutes
Ingredients:
- 1 large avocado, halved and pitted
- 2 large eggs
- 2 tomato slices, divided
- ½ cup nonfat Cottage cheese, divided
- ½ teaspoon fresh cilantro, for garnish

Directions:
1. Line the baking pan with aluminium foil.
2. Slice a thin piece from the bottom of each avocado half so they sit flat. Remove a small amount from each avocado half to make a bigger hole to hold the egg.
3. Arrange the avocado halves on the pan, hollow-side up. Break 1 egg into each half. Top each half with 1 tomato slice and ¼ cup of the Cottage cheese.
4. Slide the baking pan into Rack Position 1, select Convection Bake, set temperature to 425ºF (220ºC) and set time to 9 minutes.
5. When cooking is complete, remove the pan from the oven. Garnish with the fresh cilantro and serve.

32. Spicy Egg Casserole

Servings: 8
Cooking Time: 45 Minutes
Ingredients:
- 10 eggs
- 1 cup Colby jack cheese, shredded
- 1 cup cottage cheese
- 1 tsp baking powder
- 1/3 cup flour
- 1/2 cup milk
- 4.5 oz can green chilies, chopped
- 1/2 small onion, minced
- 2 tbsp butter
- 1 tsp seasoned salt

Directions:
1. Fit the oven with the rack in position
2. Spray 9*13-inch casserole dish with cooking spray and set aside.
3. Melt butter in a pan over medium heat.
4. Add onion and green chilies and sauté for 5 minutes. Remove pan from heat and set aside.
5. In a small bowl, whisk milk, baking powder, and flour until smooth.
6. In a mixing bowl, whisk eggs with cheese, cottage cheese, and seasoned salt.
7. Add sautéed onion and green chilies, milk, and flour mixture to the eggs and whisk until well combined.
8. Pour egg mixture into the prepared casserole dish.

9. Set to bake at 350 F for 50 minutes. After 5 minutes place the casserole dish in the preheated oven.
10. Serve and enjoy.
Nutrition Info: Calories 219 Fat 13.8 g Carbohydrates 8.4 g Sugar 1.4 g Protein 14.9 g Cholesterol 228 mg

33. Breakfast Potatoes

Servings: 4
Cooking Time: 35 Minutes
Ingredients:
- 2 lbs potatoes, scrubbed and cut into 1/2-inch cubes
- 1 tsp garlic powder
- 1 tbsp olive oil
- 1/2 tsp sweet paprika
- Pepper
- Salt

Directions:
1. Fit the oven with the rack in position
2. Place potato cubes on the parchment-lined baking pan.
3. Drizzle with oil and season with paprika, garlic powder, pepper, and salt. Toss potatoes well.
4. Set to bake at 425 F for 40 minutes, after 5 minutes, place the baking pan in the oven.
5. Serve and enjoy.
Nutrition Info: Calories 190 Fat 3.8 g Carbohydrates 36.3 g Sugar 2.8 g Protein 4 g Cholesterol 0 mg

34. Spinach Egg Breakfast

Servings: 4
Cooking Time: 20 Minutes
Ingredients:
- 3 eggs
- 1/4 cup coconut milk
- 1/4 cup parmesan cheese, grated 4 oz spinach, chopped
- 3 oz cottage cheese

Directions:
1. Preheat the air fryer to 350 F.
2. Add eggs, milk, half parmesan cheese, and cottage cheese in a bowl and whisk well. Add spinach and stir well.
3. Pour mixture into the air fryer baking dish.
4. Sprinkle remaining half parmesan cheese on top.
5. Place dish in the air fryer and cook for 20 minutes.
6. Serve and enjoy.
Nutrition Info: Calories 144 Fat 8.5 g Carbohydrates 2.5 g Sugar 1.1 g Protein 14 g Cholesterol 135 mg

35. Breakfast Oatmeal Cake

Servings: 8
Cooking Time: 25 Minutes
Ingredients:
- 2 eggs
- 1 tbsp coconut oil
- 3 tbsp yogurt
- 1/2 tsp baking powder
- 1 tsp cinnamon
- 1 tsp vanilla
- 3 tbsp honey
- 1/2 tsp baking soda
- 1 apple, peel & chopped
- 1 cup oats

Directions:
1. Fit the oven with the rack in position
2. Line baking dish with parchment paper and set aside.
3. Add 3/4 cup oats and remaining ingredients into the blender and blend until smooth.
4. Add remaining oats and stir well.
5. Pour mixture into the prepared baking dish.
6. Set to bake at 350 F for 30 minutes. After 5 minutes place the baking dish in the preheated oven.
7. Slice and serve.
Nutrition Info: Calories 114 Fat 3.6 g Carbohydrates 18.2 g Sugar 10 g Protein 3.2 g Cholesterol 41 mg

36. Olive & Tomato Tart With Feta Cheese

Servings: 2
Cooking Time: 25 Minutes
Ingredients:
- 4 eggs
- ½ cup tomatoes, chopped
- 1 cup feta cheese, crumbled
- 1 tbsp fresh basil, chopped
- 1 tbsp fresh oregano, chopped
- ¼ cup Kalamata olives, chopped
- ¼ cup onion, chopped
- 2 tbsp olive oil
- ½ cup milk
- Salt and black pepper to taste

Directions:
1. Preheat on Bake function to 360 F. Brush a pie pan with olive oil. Beat the eggs along with the milk, salt, and pepper. Stir in all of the remaining ingredients. Pour the egg mixture into the pan. Cook for 20 minutes.

37. Eggplant Hoagies

Servings: 3 Hoagies
Cooking Time: 12 Minutes
Ingredients:
- 6 peeled eggplant slices (about ½ inch thick and 3 inches in diameter)
- ¼ cup jarred pizza sauce
- 6 tablespoons grated Parmesan cheese
- 3 Italian sub rolls, split open lengthwise, warmed
- Cooking spray

Directions:
1.   Spritz the air fryer basket with cooking spray.
2.   Arrange the eggplant slices in the pan and spritz with cooking spray.
3.   Put the air fryer basket on the baking pan and slide into Rack Position 2, select Air Fry, set temperature to 350ºF (180ºC) and set time to 10 minutes.
4.   Flip the slices halfway through the cooking time.
5.   When cooked, the eggplant slices should be lightly wilted and tender.
6.   Divide and spread the pizza sauce and cheese on top of the eggplant slice
7.   Put the air fryer basket on the baking pan and slide into Rack Position 2, select Air Fry, set temperature to 375ºF (190ºC) and set time to 2 minutes.
8.   When cooked, the cheese will be melted.
9.   Assemble each sub roll with two slices of eggplant and serve immediately.

38. Maple Walnut Pancake

Servings: 4
Cooking Time: 20 Minutes
Ingredients:
- 3 tablespoons melted butter, divided
- 1 cup flour
- 2 tablespoons sugar
- 1½ teaspoons baking powder
- ¼ teaspoon salt
- 1 egg, beaten
- ¾ cup milk
- 1 teaspoon pure vanilla extract
- ½ cup roughly chopped walnuts
- Maple syrup or fresh sliced fruit, for serving

Directions:
1.   Grease the baking pan with 1 tablespoon of melted butter.
2.   Mix together the flour, sugar, baking powder, and salt in a medium bowl. Add the beaten egg, milk, the remaining 2 tablespoons of melted butter, and vanilla and stir until the batter is sticky but slightly lumpy.
3.   Slowly pour the batter into the greased baking pan and scatter with the walnuts.
4.   Slide the baking pan into Rack Position 1, select Convection Bake, set temperature to 330ºF (166ºC) and set time to 20 minutes.
5.   When cooked, the pancake should be golden brown and cooked through.
6.   Let the pancake rest for 5 minutes and serve topped with the maple syrup or fresh fruit, if desired.

39. Sausage Omelet

Servings: 2
Cooking Time: 13 Minutes
Ingredients:
- 4 eggs
- 1 bacon slice, chopped
- 2 sausages, chopped
- 1 yellow onion, chopped

Directions:
1.   In a bowl, crack the eggs and beat well.
2.   Add the remaining ingredients and gently, stir to combine.
3.   Place the mixture into a baking pan.
4.   Press "Power Button" of Air Fry Oven and turn the dial to select the "Air Fry" mode.
5.   Press the Time button and again turn the dial to set the cooking time to 13 minutes.
6.   Now push the Temp button and rotate the dial to set the temperature at 320 degrees F.
7.   Press "Start/Pause" button to start.
8.   When the unit beeps to show that it is preheated, open the lid.
9.   Arrange pan over the "Wire Rack" and insert in the oven.
10.   Cut into equal-sized wedges and serve hot.
Nutrition Info: Calories 325 Total Fat 23.1 g Saturated Fat 7.4 g Cholesterol 368 mg Sodium 678 mg Total Carbs 6 g Fiber 1.2 g Sugar 3 g Protein 22.7 g

40. Pepperoni Omelet

Servings: 2
Cooking Time: 12 Minutes
Ingredients:
- 4 eggs
- 2 tablespoons milk
- Pinch of salt
- Ground black pepper, as required
- 8-10 turkey pepperoni slices

Directions:
1.   In a bowl, crack the eggs and beat well.
2.   Add the remaining ingredients and gently, stir to combine.
3.   Place the mixture into a baking pan.

4. Press "Power Button" of Air Fry Oven and turn the dial to select the "Air Fry" mode.
5. Press the Time button and again turn the dial to set the cooking time to 12 minutes.
6. Now push the Temp button and rotate the dial to set the temperature at 355 degrees F.
7. Press "Start/Pause" button to start.
8. When the unit beeps to show that it is preheated, open the lid.
9. Arrange pan over the "Wire Rack" and insert in the oven.
10. Cut into equal-sized wedges and serve hot.
Nutrition Info: Calories 149 Total Fat 10 g Saturated Fat 3.3 g Cholesterol 337 mg Sodium 350 mg Total Carbs 1.5 g Fiber 0 g Sugar 1.4 g Protein 13.6 g

6. Press "Power Button" of Air Fry Oven and turn the dial to select the "Air Fry" mode.
7. Press the Time button and again turn the dial to set the cooking time to 10 minutes.
8. Now push the Temp button and rotate the dial to set the temperature at 355 degrees F.
9. Press "Start/Pause" button to start.
10. When the unit beeps to show that it is preheated, open the lid.
11. Arrange pan over the "Wire Rack" and insert in the oven.
12. Cut the omelet into 2 portions and serve hot.
Nutrition Info: Calories 159 Total Fat 10.9 g Saturated Fat 4 g Cholesterol 332 mg Sodium 224 mg Total Carbs 4.1 g Fiber 1.1 g Sugar 2.4 g Protein 12.3 g

41. Buttered Apple & Brie Cheese Sandwich

Servings: 1
Cooking Time: 10 Minutes
Ingredients:
- 2 bread slices
- ½ apple, thinly sliced
- 2 tsp butter
- 2 oz brie cheese, thinly sliced

Directions:
1. Spread butter on the bread slices. Top with apple slices. Place brie slices on top of the apples. Finish with the other slice of bread. Cook in for 5 minutes at 350 F on Bake function.

42. Zucchini Omelet

Servings: 2
Cooking Time: 14 Minutes
Ingredients:
- 1 teaspoon butter
- 1 zucchini, julienned
- 4 eggs
- ¼ teaspoon fresh basil, chopped
- ¼ teaspoon red pepper flakes, crushed
- Salt and ground black pepper, as required

Directions:
1. In a skillet, melt the butter over medium heat and cook the zucchini for about 3-4 minutes.
2. Remove from the heat and set aside to cool slightly.
3. Meanwhile, in a bowl, mix together the eggs, basil, red pepper flakes, salt, and black pepper.
4. Add the cooked zucchini and gently, stir to combine.
5. Place the zucchini mixture into a small baking pan.

43. Baked Eggs

Servings: 4
Cooking Time: 15-20 | Minutes
Ingredients:
- 7 Oz. leg ham
- 4 eggs
- 4 tsps full cream milk Margarine
- 1 lb baby spinach
- 1 tablespoon olive oil Salt and Pepper to taste

Directions:
1. Preheat the Air Fryer to 350°F. Layer four ramekins with margarine.
2. Equally divide the spinach and ham into the four ramekins. Break 1 egg into each and add a tsp. of milk. Spice with salt and pepper.
3. Place into Air Fryer for about 15-20 minutes. For a runny yolk, cook for 15 minutes, for fully cooked; 20 minutes.
Nutrition Info: Calories 113 Fat 8.2 g Carbohydrates 0.3 g Sugar 0.2 g Protein 5.4 g Cholesterol 18 mg

44. Lemon Cupcakes With Orange Frosting

Servings: 4
Cooking Time: 30 Minutes
Ingredients:
- Orange Frosting:
- 1 cup plain yogurt
- 2 tbsp sugar
- 1 orange, juiced and juiced
- 1 cup cream cheese
- Cupcake:
- 2 lemons, quartered and seeded
- ½ cup flour + extra for basing
- ¼ tsp salt

- 2 tbsp sugar
- 1 tsp baking powder
- 1 tsp vanilla extract
- 2 eggs
- ½ cup softened butter
- 2 tbsp milk

Directions:

1. In a bowl, mix the yogurt and cream cheese. Stir in the orange juice and zest. Gradually add the sugar while stirring until smooth. Make sure the frost is not runny. Set aside.
2. Place the lemon quarters in a food processor and process until pureed. Add in baking powder, softened butter, milk, eggs, vanilla extract, sugar, and salt. Process again until smooth.
3. Preheat Breville on Bake function to 400 F. Flour the bottom of 8 cupcake cases and spoon the batter into the cases ¾ way up. Place them in a baking tray and press Start. Bake for 20 minutes. Remove and let cool. Design the cupcakes with the frosting to serve.

45. Tomatta Spinacha Frittata

Servings: 4
Cooking Time: 30 Minutes
Ingredients:

- 3 tablespoons olive oil
- 10 large eggs
- 2 teaspoons kosher salt
- 1/2 teaspoon black pepper
- 1 (5-ounce) bag baby spinach
- 1 pint grape tomatoes
- 4 scallions
- 8 ounces feta cheese

Directions:

1. Preheat toaster oven to 350°F.
2. Halve tomatoes and slice scallions into thin pieces.
3. Add oil to a 2-quart oven-safe pan, making sure to brush it on the sides as well as the bottom. Place the dish in toaster oven.
4. Combine the eggs, salt, and pepper in a medium mixing bowl and whisk together for a minute.
5. Add spinach, tomatoes, and scallions to the bowl and mix together until even.
6. Crumble feta cheese into the bowl and mix together gently. Remove the dish from the oven and pour in the egg mixture.
7. Put the dish back into the oven and bake for 25–30 minutes, or until the edges of the frittata are browned.

Nutrition Info: Calories: 448, Sodium: 515 mg, Dietary Fiber: 2.3 g, Total Fat: 35.4 g, Total Carbs: 9.3 g, Protein: 25.9 g.

46. Banana Oat Muffins

Servings: 6
Cooking Time: 25 Minutes
Ingredients:

- 1 egg
- 2 tbsp butter, melted
- 1/2 tsp cinnamon
- 1 tsp vanilla
- 2 tbsp yogurt
- 1 1/2 cup oats
- 1 tsp baking powder
- 2 ripe bananas, mashed

Directions:

1. Fit the oven with the rack in position
2. Line the muffin tray with cupcake liners and set aside.
3. In a bowl, whisk the egg with banana, yogurt, vanilla, cinnamon, baking powder, and butter.
4. Add oats and mix well.
5. Pour mixture into the prepared muffin tray.
6. Set to bake at 350 F for 30 minutes. After 5 minutes place the muffin tray in the preheated oven.
7. Serve and enjoy.

Nutrition Info: Calories 164 Fat 6.1 g Carbohydrates 23.9 g Sugar 5.5 g Protein 4.4 g Cholesterol 38 mg

47. Prosciutto & Salami Egg Bake

Servings: 2
Cooking Time: 20 Minutes
Ingredients:

- 1 beef sausage, chopped
- 4 slices prosciutto, chopped
- 3 oz salami, chopped
- 1 cup grated mozzarella cheese
- 4 eggs, beaten
- ½ tsp onion powder

Directions:

1. Preheat on Bake function to 350 F. Whisk the eggs with the onion powder. Brown the sausage in a skillet over medium heat for 2 minutes. Remove to the egg mixture and add in mozzarella cheese, salami, and prosciutto and give it a stir. Pour the egg mixture in a greased baking pan and cook for 10-15 minutes until golden brown on top. Serve.

48. Spiced Squash Mix

Servings: 4
Cooking Time: 15 Minutes
Ingredients:

- 1 cup almond milk
- 1 butternut squash, peeled and roughly cubed
- ½ teaspoon cinnamon powder
- ¼ teaspoon nutmeg, ground

- ¼ teaspoon allspice, ground
- ¼ teaspoon cardamom, ground
- 2 tablespoons brown sugar
- Cooking spray

Directions:
1. Spray your air fryer with cooking spray, add the squash, milk and the other ingredients, toss, cover and cook at 360 degrees F for 15 minutes.
2. Divide into bowls and serve for breakfast.

Nutrition Info: calories 212, fat 5, fiber 7, carbs 14, protein 5

49. Sweet Berry Pastry

Servings: 3
Cooking Time: 20 Minutes
Ingredients:
- 3 pastry dough sheets
- 2 tbsp strawberries, mashed
- 2 tbsp raspberries, mashed
- ¼ tsp vanilla extract
- 2 cups cream cheese, softened
- 1 tbsp honey

Directions:
1. Preheat Breville oven on Bake function to 375 F. Spread the cream cheese on the dough sheets. In a bowl, combine berries, honey, and vanilla. Divide the mixture between the pastry sheets. Pinch the ends of the sheets to form puff. Place in the Breville oven and cook for 15 minutes.

50. Cheesy Potato & Spinach Frittata

Servings: 4
Cooking Time: 35 Minutes
Ingredients:
- 3 cups potato cubes, boiled
- 2 cups spinach, chopped
- 5 eggs, lightly beaten
- ¼ cup heavy cream
- 1 cup grated mozzarella cheese
- ½ cup parsley, chopped
- Fresh thyme, chopped
- Salt and black pepper to taste

Directions:
1. Spray the Air Fryer tray with oil. Arrange the potatoes inside.
2. In a bowl, whisk eggs, cream, spinach, mozzarella, parsley, thyme, salt and pepper, and pour over the potatoes. Cook in your for 16 minutes at 360 F on Bake function until nice and golden. Serve sliced.

51. Sweet Potato And Black Bean Burritos

Servings: 6 Burritos

Cooking Time: 30 Minutes
Ingredients:
- 2 sweet potatoes, peeled and cut into a small dice
- 1 tablespoon vegetable oil
- Kosher salt and ground black pepper, to taste
- 6 large flour tortillas
- 1 (16-ounce / 454-g) can refried black beans, divided
- 1½ cups baby spinach, divided
- 6 eggs, scrambled
- ¾ cup grated Cheddar cheese, divided
- ¼ cup salsa
- ¼ cup sour cream
- Cooking spray

Directions:
1. Put the sweet potatoes in a large bowl, then drizzle with vegetable oil and sprinkle with salt and black pepper. Toss to coat well.
2. Place the potatoes in the air fryer basket.
3. Put the air fryer basket on the baking pan and slide into Rack Position 2, select Air Fry, set temperature to 400ºF (205ºC) and set time to 10 minutes.
4. Flip the potatoes halfway through the cooking time.
5. When done, the potatoes should be lightly browned. Remove the potatoes from the oven.
6. Unfold the tortillas on a clean work surface. Divide the black beans, spinach, air fried sweet potatoes, scrambled eggs, and cheese on top of the tortillas.
7. Fold the long side of the tortillas over the filling, then fold in the shorter side to wrap the filling to make the burritos.
8. Wrap the burritos in the aluminum foil and put in the pan.
9. Put the air fryer basket on the baking pan and slide into Rack Position 2, select Air Fry, set temperature to 350ºF (180ºC) and set time to 20 minutes.
10. Flip the burritos halfway through the cooking time.
11. Remove the burritos from the oven and spread with sour cream and salsa. Serve immediately.

52. Feta & Egg Rolls

Servings: 4
Cooking Time: 50 Minutes
Ingredients:
- 1 cup feta cheese, crumbled
- 2 tbsp olive oil
- 4 eggs, beaten
- 5 sheets frozen filo pastry, thawed

Directions:

1. Gently unroll the filo sheets. Brush them with olive oil. In a bowl, mix feta cheese and eggs, and parsley. Divide the feta mixture between the sheets.
2. Using your fingers, roll them upwards like a long sausage. Place the rolls in a greased baking dish and cook in the Breville oven for 30-35 minutes at 360 F on Bake function. Serve warm.

53. Flavorful Zucchini Frittata

Servings: 4
Cooking Time: 25 Minutes
Ingredients:
- 6 eggs
- 2 cups zucchini, grated & squeeze out excess liquid
- 1 cup cheddar cheese, shredded
- 1 cup ham, chopped
- 1/4 cup heavy cream
- 2 tbsp butter
- 1/4 tsp pepper
- 1 tsp salt

Directions:
1. Fit the oven with the rack in position
2. Melt butter in a pan over medium heat.
3. Add zucchini in the pan and sauté until tender. Remove pan from heat.
4. In a bowl, whisk eggs and cream. Stir in zucchini, cheese, ham, pepper, and salt.
5. Pour mixture into the greased baking dish.
6. Set to bake at 325 F for 30 minutes. After 5 minutes place the baking dish in the preheated oven.
7. Serve and enjoy.

Nutrition Info: Calories 349 Fat 27.5 g Carbohydrates 4.3 g Sugar 1.7 g Protein 21.8 gCholesterol 320 mg

54. Buttery Cheese Sandwich

Servings: 1
Cooking Time: 10 Minutes
Ingredients:
- 2 tbsp butter
- 2 slices bread
- 3 slices American cheese

Directions:
1. Preheat on Bake function to 370 F. Spread one tsp of butter on the outside of each of the bread slices. Place the cheese on the inside of one bread slice. Top with the other slice. Cook in the toaster oven for 4 minutes. Flip the sandwich over and cook for an additional 4 minutes. Serve sliced diagonally.

55. Banana & Peanut Butter Cake

Servings: 4
Cooking Time: 30 Minutes
Ingredients:
- 1 cup flour
- ¼ tsp baking soda
- 1 tsp baking powder
- ⅓ cup sugar
- 2 mashed bananas
- ¼ cup vegetable oil
- 1 egg, beaten
- 1 tsp vanilla extract
- ¾ cup chopped walnuts
- ¼ tsp salt
- 2 tbsp peanut butter
- 2 tbsp sour cream

Directions:
1. Preheat on Bake function to 350 F. Spray a 9-inch baking pan with cooking spray or grease with butter. Combine the flour, salt, baking powder, and baking soda in a bowl.
2. In another bowl, combine bananas, oil, egg, peanut butter, vanilla, sugar, and sour cream. Combine both mixtures gently. Stir in the chopped walnuts. Pour the batter into the pan. Cook for 20 minutes. Let cool completely and serve sliced.

56. Quick Paprika Eggs

Servings: 4
Cooking Time: 10 Minutes
Ingredients:
- 4 large eggs
- 1 tsp paprika
- Salt and pepper to taste
- ¼ cup cottage cheese, crumbled

Directions:
1. Preheat your fryer to 350 F on Bake function. Crack an egg into a muffin cup. Repeat with the remaining cups. Sprinkle with salt and pepper. Top with cottage cheese. Put the cups in the Air Fryer tray and bake for 8-10 minutes. Remove and sprinkle with paprika to serve.

57. Avocado And Spinach With Poached Eggs

Servings: 1
Cooking Time: 10 Minutes
Ingredients:
- 2 eggs
- 1/2 avocado
- 2 slices bread
- 1 bunch spinach

- Pinch of salt
- Pinch of pepper

Directions:

1. Start by preheating toaster oven to 400°F.
2. Bring a pan of water to a rolling boil.
3. Place bread on a pan and toast it in the oven for 10 minutes.
4. Once the water is boiling, whisk it around in a circle until it creates a vortex.
5. Drop one egg in the hole and turn the heat to low, then poach for 2 minutes.
6. Repeat with the second egg.
7. Mash avocado and spread it over the toast while the eggs poach.
8. Add the eggs to the toast and top with spinach.

Nutrition Info: Calories: 409, Sodium: 553 mg, Dietary Fiber: 14.2 g, Total Fat: 29.7 g, Total Carbs: 21.7 g, Protein: 22.7 g.

LUNCH RECIPES

58. Simple Turkey Breast

Servings: 10
Cooking Time: 40 Minutes
Ingredients:
- 1: 8-poundsbone-in turkey breast
- Salt and black pepper, as required
- 2 tablespoons olive oil

Directions:
1. Preheat the Air fryer to 360 degree F and grease an Air fryer basket.
2. Season the turkey breast with salt and black pepper and drizzle with oil.
3. Arrange the turkey breast into the Air Fryer basket, skin side down and cook for about 20 minutes.
4. Flip the side and cook for another 20 minutes.
5. Dish out in a platter and cut into desired size slices to serve.

Nutrition Info: Calories: 719, Fat: 35.9g, Carbohydrates: 0g, Sugar: 0g, Protein: 97.2g, Sodium: 386mg

59. Easy Prosciutto Grilled Cheese

Servings: 1
Cooking Time: 5 Minutes
Ingredients:
- 2 slices muenster cheese
- 2 slices white bread
- Four thinly-shaved pieces of prosciutto
- 1 tablespoon sweet and spicy pickles

Directions:
1. Set toaster oven to the Toast setting.
2. Place one slice of cheese on each piece of bread.
3. Put prosciutto on one slice and pickles on the other.
4. Transfer to a baking sheet and toast for 4 minutes or until the cheese is melted.
5. Combine the sides, cut, and serve.

Nutrition Info: Calories: 460, Sodium: 2180 mg, Dietary Fiber: 0 g, Total Fat: 25.2 g, Total Carbs: 11.9 g, Protein: 44.2 g.

60. Basic Roasted Tofu

Servings: 4
Cooking Time: 45 Minutes
Ingredients:
- 1 or more (16-ounce) containers extra-firm tofu
- 1 tablespoon sesame oil
- 1 tablespoon soy sauce
- 1 tablespoon rice vinegar
- 1 tablespoon water

Directions:
1. Start by drying the tofu: first pat dry with paper towels, then lay on another set of paper towels or a dish towel.
2. Put a plate on top of the tofu then put something heavy on the plate (like a large can of vegetables). Leave it there for at least 20 minutes.
3. While tofu is being pressed, whip up marinade by combining oil, soy sauce, vinegar, and water in a bowl and set aside.
4. Cut the tofu into squares or sticks. Place the tofu in the marinade for at least 30 minutes.
5. Preheat toaster oven to 350°F. Line a pan with parchment paper and add as many pieces of tofu as you can, giving each piece adequate space.
6. Bake 20–45 minutes; tofu is done when the outside edges look golden brown. Time will vary depending on tofu size and shape.

Nutrition Info: Calories: 114, Sodium: 239 mg, Dietary Fiber: 1.1 g, Total Fat: 8.1 g, Total Carbs: 2.2 g, Protein: 9.5 g.

61. Bbq Chicken Breasts

Servings: 4
Cooking Time: 15 Minutes
Ingredients:
- 4 boneless skinless chicken breast about 6 oz each
- 1-2 Tbsp bbq seasoning

Directions:
1. Cover both sides of chicken breast with the BBQ seasoning. Cover and marinate the in the refrigerator for 45 minutes.
2. Choose the Air Fry option and set the temperature to 400°F. Push start and let it preheat for 5 minutes.
3. Upon preheating, place the chicken breast in the Instant Pot Duo Crisp Air Fryer basket, making sure they do not overlap. Spray with oil.
4. Cook for 13-14 minutes
5. flipping halfway.
6. Remove chicken when the chicken reaches an internal temperature of 160°F. Place on a plate and allow to rest for 5 minutes before slicing.

Nutrition Info: Calories 131, Total Fat 3g, Total Carbs 2g, Protein 24g

62. Tomato And Avocado

Servings: 4
Cooking Time: 12 Minutes
Ingredients:
- ½ lb. cherry tomatoes; halved

- 2 avocados, pitted; peeled and cubed
- 1 ¼ cup lettuce; torn
- 1/3 cup coconut cream
- A pinch of salt and black pepper
- Cooking spray

Directions:
1. Grease the air fryer with cooking spray, combine the tomatoes with avocados, salt, pepper and the cream and cook at 350°F for 5 minutes shaking once
2. In a salad bowl, mix the lettuce with the tomatoes and avocado mix, toss and serve.

Nutrition Info: Calories: 226; Fat: 12g; Fiber: 2g; Carbs: 4g; Protein: 8g

63. Lemon Pepper Turkey

Servings: 6
Cooking Time: 45 Minutes
Ingredients:
- 3 lbs. turkey breast
- 2 tablespoons oil
- 1 tablespoon Worcestershire sauce
- 1 teaspoon lemon pepper
- 1/2 teaspoon salt

Directions:
1. Whisk everything in a bowl and coat the turkey liberally.
2. Place the turkey in the Air fryer basket.
3. Press "Power Button" of Air Fry Oven and turn the dial to select the "Air Fry" mode.
4. Press the Time button and again turn the dial to set the cooking time to 45 minutes.
5. Now push the Temp button and rotate the dial to set the temperature at 375 degrees F.
6. Once preheated, place the air fryer basket inside and close its lid.
7. Serve warm.

Nutrition Info: Calories 391 Total Fat 2.8 g Saturated Fat 0.6 g Cholesterol 330 mg Sodium 62 mg Total Carbs 36.5 g Fiber 9.2 g Sugar 4.5 g Protein 6.6

64. Chicken Parmesan

Servings: 4
Cooking Time: 10 Minutes
Ingredients:
- 2 (6-oz.boneless, skinless chicken breasts
- 1 oz. pork rinds, crushed
- ½ cup grated Parmesan cheese, divided.
- 1 cup low-carb, no-sugar-added pasta sauce.
- 1 cup shredded mozzarella cheese, divided.
- 4 tbsp. full-fat mayonnaise, divided.
- ½ tsp. garlic powder.
- ¼ tsp. dried oregano.

- ½ tsp. dried parsley.

Directions:
1. Slice each chicken breast in half lengthwise and lb. out to 3/4-inch thickness. Sprinkle with garlic powder, oregano and parsley
2. Spread 1 tbsp. mayonnaise on top of each piece of chicken, then sprinkle ¼ cup mozzarella on each piece.
3. In a small bowl, mix the crushed pork rinds and Parmesan. Sprinkle the mixture on top of mozzarella
4. Pour sauce into 6-inch round baking pan and place chicken on top. Place pan into the air fryer basket. Adjust the temperature to 320 Degrees F and set the timer for 25 minutes
5. Cheese will be browned and internal temperature of the chicken will be at least 165 Degrees F when fully cooked. Serve warm.

Nutrition Info: Calories: 393; Protein: 32g; Fiber: 1g; Fat: 28g; Carbs: 8g

65. Carrot And Beef Cocktail Balls

Servings: 10
Cooking Time: 20 Minutes
Ingredients:
- 1-pound ground beef
- 2 carrots
- 1 red onion, peeled and chopped
- 2 cloves garlic
- 1/2 teaspoon dried rosemary, crushed
- 1/2 teaspoon dried basil
- 1 teaspoon dried oregano
- 1 egg
- 3/4 cup breadcrumbs
- 1/2 teaspoon salt
- 1/2 teaspoon black pepper, or to taste
- 1 cup plain flour

Directions:
1. Preparing the ingredients. Place ground beef in a large bowl.
2. In a food processor, pulse the carrot, onion and garlic; transfer the vegetable mixture to a large-sized bowl.
3. Then, add the rosemary, basil, oregano, egg, breadcrumbs, salt, and black pepper.
4. Shape the mixture into even balls; refrigerate for about 30 minutes.
5. Roll the balls into the flour.
6. Air frying. Close air fryer lid.
7. Then, air-fry the balls at 350 degrees f for about 20 minutes, turning occasionally; work with batches. Serve with toothpicks.

Nutrition Info: Calories 284 Total fat 7.9 g Saturated fat 1.4 g Cholesterol 36 mg Sodium 704 mg Total carbs 46 g Fiber 3.6 g Sugar 5.5 g Protein 17.9 g

66. Chili Chicken Sliders

Servings: 4
Cooking Time: 10 Minutes
Ingredients:
- 1/3 teaspoon paprika
- 1/3 cup scallions, peeled and chopped
- 3 cloves garlic, peeled and minced
- 1 teaspoon ground black pepper, or to taste
- 1/2 teaspoon fresh basil, minced
- 1 ½ cups chicken,minced
- 1 ½ tablespoons coconut aminos
- 1/2 teaspoon grated fresh ginger
- 1/2 tablespoon chili sauce
- 1 teaspoon salt

Directions:
1. Thoroughly combine all ingredients in a mixing dish. Then, form into 4 patties.
2. Cook in the preheated Air Fryer for 18 minutes at 355 degrees F.
3. Garnish with toppings of choice.

Nutrition Info: 366 Calories; 6g Fat; 4g Carbs; 66g Protein; 3g Sugars; 9g Fiber

67. Cheese-stuffed Meatballs

Servings: 4
Cooking Time: 10 Minutes
Ingredients:
- ⅓ cup soft bread crumbs
- 3 tablespoons milk
- 1 tablespoon ketchup
- 1 egg
- ½ teaspoon dried marjoram
- Pinch salt
- Freshly ground black pepper
- 1-pound 95 percent lean ground beef
- 20 ½-inch cubes of cheese
- Olive oil for misting

Directions:
1. Preparing the ingredients. In a large bowl, combine the bread crumbs, milk, ketchup, egg, marjoram, salt, and pepper, and mix well. Add the ground beef and mix gently but thoroughly with your hands. Form the mixture into 20 meatballs. Shape each meatball around a cheese cube. Mist the meatballs with olive oil and put into the instant crisp air fryer basket.
2. Air frying. Close air fryer lid. Bake for 10 to 13 minutes or until the meatballs register 165°f on a meat thermometer.

Nutrition Info: Calories: 393; Fat: 17g; Protein:50g; Fiber:0g

68. Buttered Duck Breasts

Servings: 4
Cooking Time: 22 Minutes
Ingredients:
- 2: 12-ouncesduck breasts
- 3 tablespoons unsalted butter, melted
- Salt and ground black pepper, as required
- ½ teaspoon dried thyme, crushed
- ¼ teaspoon star anise powder

Directions:
1. Preheat the Air fryer to 390 degree F and grease an Air fryer basket.
2. Season the duck breasts generously with salt and black pepper.
3. Arrange the duck breasts into the prepared Air fryer basket and cook for about 10 minutes.
4. Dish out the duck breasts and drizzle with melted butter.
5. Season with thyme and star anise powder and place the duck breasts again into the Air fryer basket.
6. Cook for about 12 more minutes and dish out to serve warm.

Nutrition Info: Calories: 296, Fat: 15.5g, Carbohydrates: 0.1g, Sugar: 0g, Protein: 37.5g, Sodium: 100mg

69. Turkey And Mushroom Stew

Servings: 4
Cooking Time: 12 Minutes
Ingredients:
- ½ lb. brown mushrooms; sliced
- 1 turkey breast, skinless, boneless; cubed and browned
- ¼ cup tomato sauce
- 1 tbsp. parsley; chopped.
- Salt and black pepper to taste.

Directions:
1. In a pan that fits your air fryer, mix the turkey with the mushrooms, salt, pepper and tomato sauce, toss, introduce in the fryer and cook at 350°F for 25 minutes
2. Divide into bowls and serve for lunch with parsley sprinkled on top.

Nutrition Info: Calories: 220; Fat: 12g; Fiber: 2g; Carbs: 5g; Protein: 12g

70. Coconut Shrimp With Dip

Servings: 4
Cooking Time: 9 Minutes
Ingredients:
- 1 lb large raw shrimp peeled and deveined with tail on
- 2 eggs beaten

- ¼ cup Panko Breadcrumbs
- 1 tsp salt
- ¼ tsp black pepper
- ½ cup All-Purpose Flour
- ½ cup unsweetened shredded coconut
- Oil for spraying

Directions:
1. Clean and dry the shrimp. Set it aside.
2. Take 3 bowls. Put flour in the first bowl. Beat eggs in the second bowl. Mix coconut, breadcrumbs, salt, and black pepper in the third bowl.
3. Select the Air Fry option and adjust the temperature to 390°F. Push start and preheating will start.
4. Dip each shrimp in flour followed by the egg and then coconut mixture, ensuring shrimp is covered on all sides during each dip.
5. Once the preheating is done, place shrimp in a single layer on greased tray in the basket of the Instant Pot Duo Crisp Air Fryer.
6. Spray the shrimp with oil lightly, and then close the Air Fryer basket lid. Cook for around 4 minutes.
7. After 4 minutes
8. open the Air Fryer basket lid and flip the shrimp over. Respray the shrimp with oil, close the Air Fryer basket lid, and cook for five more minutes.
9. Remove shrimp from the basket and serve with Thai Sweet Chili Sauce.

Nutrition Info: Calories 279, Total Fat 11g, Total Carbs 17g, Protein 28g

71. Coriander Potatoes

Servings: 4
Cooking Time: 25 Minutes
Ingredients:
- 1 pound gold potatoes, peeled and cut into wedges
- Salt and black pepper to the taste
- 1 tablespoon tomato sauce
- 2 tablespoons coriander, chopped
- ½ teaspoon garlic powder
- 1 teaspoon chili powder
- 1 tablespoon olive oil

Directions:
1. In a bowl, combine the potatoes with the tomato sauce and the other Ingredients:, toss, and transfer to the air fryer's basket.
2. Cook at 370 degrees F for 25 minutes, divide between plates and serve as a side dish.

Nutrition Info: Calories 210, fat 5, fiber 7, carbs 12, protein 5

72. Barbecue Air Fried Chicken

Servings: 10
Cooking Time: 26 Minutes
Ingredients:
- 1 teaspoon Liquid Smoke
- 2 cloves Fresh Garlic smashed
- 1/2 cup Apple Cider Vinegar
- 3 pounds Chuck Roast well-marbled with intramuscular fat
- 1 Tablespoon Kosher Salt
- 1 Tablespoon Freshly Ground Black Pepper
- 2 teaspoons Garlic Powder
- 1.5 cups Barbecue Sauce
- 1/4 cup Light Brown Sugar + more for sprinkling
- 2 Tablespoons Honey optional and in place of 2 TBL sugar

Directions:
1. Add meat to the Instant Pot Duo Crisp Air Fryer Basket, spreading out the meat.
2. Select the option Air Fry.
3. Close the Air Fryer lid and cook at 300 degrees F for 8 minutes. Pause the Air Fryer and flip meat over after 4 minutes.
4. Remove the lid and baste with more barbecue sauce and sprinkle with a little brown sugar.
5. Again Close the Air Fryer lid and set the temperature at 400°F for 9 minutes. Watch meat though the lid and flip it over after 5 minutes.

Nutrition Info: Calories 360, Total Fat 16g, Total Carbs 27g, Protein 27g

73. Deviled Chicken

Servings: 8
Cooking Time: 40 Minutes
Ingredients:
- 2 tablespoons butter
- 2 cloves garlic, chopped
- 1 cup Dijon mustard
- 1/2 teaspoon cayenne pepper
- 1 1/2 cups panko breadcrumbs
- 3/4 cup Parmesan, freshly grated
- 1/4 cup chives, chopped
- 2 teaspoons paprika
- 8 small bone-in chicken thighs, skin removed

Directions:
1. Toss the chicken thighs with crumbs, cheese, chives, butter, and spices in a bowl and mix well to coat.
2. Transfer the chicken along with its spice mix to a baking pan.
3. Press "Power Button" of Air Fry Oven and turn the dial to select the "Air Fry" mode.

4. Press the Time button and again turn the dial to set the cooking time to 40 minutes.
5. Now push the Temp button and rotate the dial to set the temperature at 350 degrees F.
6. Once preheated, place the baking pan inside and close its lid.
7. Serve warm.
Nutrition Info: Calories 380 Total Fat 20 g Saturated Fat 5 g Cholesterol 151 mg Sodium 686 mg Total Carbs 33 g Fiber 1 g Sugar 1.2 g Protein 21 g

74. Amazing Mac And Cheese

Servings:
Cooking Time: 12 Minutes
Ingredients:
- 1 cup cooked macaroni
- 1/2 cup warm milk
- 1 tablespoon parmesan cheese
- 1 cup grated cheddar cheese
- salt and pepper; to taste
Directions:
1. Preheat the Air Fryer to 350 - degrees Fahrenheit. Stir all of the ingredients; except Parmesan, in a baking dish.
2. Place the dish inside the Air Fryer and cook for 10 minutes. Top with the Parmesan cheese.

75. Air Fried Steak Sandwich

Servings: 4
Cooking Time: 16 Minutes
Ingredients:
- Large hoagie bun, sliced in half
- 6 ounces of sirloin or flank steak, sliced into bite-sized pieces
- ½ tablespoon of mustard powder
- ½ tablespoon of soy sauce
- 1 tablespoon of fresh bleu cheese, crumbled
- 8 medium-sized cherry tomatoes, sliced in half
- 1 cup of fresh arugula, rinsed and patted dry
Directions:
1. Preparing the ingredients. In a small mixing bowl, combine the soy sauce and onion powder; stir with a fork until thoroughly combined.
2. Lay the raw steak strips in the soy-mustard mixture, and fully immerse each piece to marinate.
3. Set the instant crisp air fryer to 320 degrees for 10 minutes.
4. Arrange the soy-mustard marinated steak pieces on a piece of tin foil, flat and not overlapping, and set the tin foil on one side of the instant crisp air fryer basket. The foil should not take up more than half of the surface.

5. Lay the hoagie-bun halves, crusty-side up and soft-side down, on the other half of the air-fryer.
6. Air frying. Close air fryer lid.
7. After 10 minutes, the instant crisp air fryer will shut off; the hoagie buns should be starting to crisp and the steak will have begun to cook.
8. Carefully, flip the hoagie buns so they are now crusty-side down and soft-side up; crumble a layer of the bleu cheese on each hoagie half.
9. With a long spoon, gently stir the marinated steak in the foil to ensure even coverage.
10. Set the instant crisp air fryer to 360 degrees for 6 minutes.
11. After 6 minutes, when the fryer shuts off, the bleu cheese will be perfectly melted over the toasted bread, and the steak will be juicy on the inside and crispy on the outside.
12. Remove the cheesy hoagie halves first, using tongs, and set on a serving plate; then cover one side with the steak, and top with the cherry-tomato halves and the arugula. Close with the other cheesy hoagie-half, slice into two pieces, and enjoy.
Nutrition Info: Calories 284 Total fat 7.9 g Saturated fat 1.4 g Cholesterol 36 mg Sodium 704 mg Total carbs 46 g Fiber 3.6 g Sugar 5.5 g Protein 17.9 g

76. Sweet Potato And Eggplant Mix

Servings: 4
Cooking Time: 20 Minutes
Ingredients:
- 2 sweet potatoes, peeled and cut into medium wedges
- 2 eggplants, roughly cubed
- 1 tablespoon avocado oil
- Juice of 1 lemon
- 4 garlic cloves, minced
- 1 teaspoon nutmeg, ground
- Salt and black pepper to the taste
- 1 tablespoon rosemary, chopped
Directions:
1. In your air fryer, combine the potatoes with the eggplants and the other Ingredients:, toss and cook at 370 degrees F for 20 minutes.
2. Divide the mix between plates and serve as a side dish.
Nutrition Info: Calories 182, fat 6, fiber 3, carbs 11, protein 5

77. Bok Choy And Butter Sauce(1)

Servings: 4
Cooking Time: 12 Minutes
Ingredients:
- 2 bok choy heads; trimmed and cut into strips

- 1 tbsp. butter; melted
- 2 tbsp. chicken stock
- 1 tsp. lemon juice
- 1 tbsp. olive oil
- A pinch of salt and black pepper

Directions:
1. In a pan that fits your air fryer, mix all the ingredients, toss, introduce the pan in the air fryer and cook at 380°F for 15 minutes.
2. Divide between plates and serve as a side dish

Nutrition Info: Calories: 141; Fat: 3g; Fiber: 2g; Carbs: 4g; Protein: 3g

78. Herb-roasted Turkey Breast

Servings: 8
Cooking Time: 60 Minutes
Ingredients:
- 3 lb turkey breast
- Rub Ingredients:
- 2 tbsp olive oil
- 2 tbsp lemon juice
- 1 tbsp minced Garlic
- 2 tsp ground mustard
- 2 tsp kosher salt
- 1 tsp pepper
- 1 tsp dried rosemary
- 1 tsp dried thyme
- 1 tsp ground sage

Directions:
1. Take a small bowl and thoroughly combine the Rub Ingredients: in it. Rub this on the outside of the turkey breast and under any loose skin.
2. Place the coated turkey breast keeping skin side up on a cooking tray.
3. Place the drip pan at the bottom of the cooking chamber of the Instant Pot Duo Crisp Air Fryer. Select Air Fry option, post this, adjust the temperature to 360°F and the time to one hour, then touch start.
4. When preheated, add the food to the cooking tray in the lowest position. Close the lid for cooking.
5. When the Air Fry program is complete, check to make sure that the thickest portion of the meat reads at least 160°F, remove the turkey and let it rest for 10 minutes before slicing and serving.

Nutrition Info: Calories 214, Total Fat 10g, Total Carbs 2g, Protein 29g

79. Parmigiano Reggiano And Prosciutto Toasts With Balsamic Glaze

Servings: 8
Cooking Time: 15 Minutes
Ingredients:
- 3 ounces thinly sliced prosciutto, cut crosswise into 1/4-inch-wide strips
- 1 (3-ounce) piece Parmigiano Reggiano cheese
- 1/2 cup balsamic vinegar
- 1 medium red onion, thinly sliced
- 1 loaf ciabatta, cut into 3/4-inch-thick slices
- 1 tablespoon extra-virgin olive oil
- 1 clove garlic
- Black pepper to taste

Directions:
1. Preheat toaster oven to 350°F.
2. Place onion in a bowl of cold water and let sit for 10 minutes.
3. Bring vinegar to a boil, then reduce heat and simmer for 5 minutes.
4. Remove from heat completely and set aside to allow the vinegar to thicken.
5. Drain the onion.
6. Brush the tops of each bun with oil, rub with garlic, and sprinkle with pepper.
7. Use a vegetable peeler to make large curls of Parmigiano Reggiano cheese and place them on the bun.
8. Bake for 15 minutes or until the bread just starts to crisp.
9. Sprinkle prosciutto and onions on top, then drizzle vinegar and serve.

Nutrition Info: Calories: 154, Sodium: 432 mg, Dietary Fiber: 1.0 g, Total Fat: 5.6 g, Total Carbs: 17.3 g, Protein: 8.1 g.

80. Chives Radishes

Servings: 4
Cooking Time: 12 Minutes
Ingredients:
- 20 radishes; halved
- 2 tbsp. olive oil
- 1 tbsp. garlic; minced
- 1 tsp. chives; chopped.
- Salt and black pepper to taste.

Directions:
1. In your air fryer's pan, combine all the ingredients and toss.
2. Introduce the pan in the machine and cook at 370°F for 15 minutes
3. Divide between plates and serve as a side dish.

Nutrition Info: Calories: 160; Fat: 2g; Fiber: 3g; Carbs: 4g; Protein: 6g

81. Maple Chicken Thighs

Servings: 4
Cooking Time: 30 Minutes
Ingredients:

- 4 large chicken thighs, bone-in
- 2 tablespoons French mustard
- 2 tablespoons Dijon mustard
- 1 clove minced garlic
- 1/2 teaspoon dried marjoram
- 2 tablespoons maple syrup

Directions:
1. Mix chicken with everything in a bowl and coat it well.
2. Place the chicken along with its marinade in the baking pan.
3. Press "Power Button" of Air Fry Oven and turn the dial to select the "Bake" mode.
4. Press the Time button and again turn the dial to set the cooking time to 30 minutes.
5. Now push the Temp button and rotate the dial to set the temperature at 370 degrees F.
6. Once preheated, place the baking pan inside and close its lid.
7. Serve warm.

Nutrition Info: Calories 301 Total Fat 15.8 g Saturated Fat 2.7 g Cholesterol 75 mg Sodium 189 mg Total Carbs 31.7 g Fiber 0.3 g Sugar 0.1 g Protein 28.2 g

82. Boneless Air Fryer Turkey Breasts

Servings: 4
Cooking Time: 50 Minutes
Ingredients:
- 3 lb boneless breast
- ¼ cup mayonnaise
- 2 tsp poultry seasoning
- 1 tsp salt
- ½ tsp garlic powder
- ¼ tsp black pepper

Directions:
1. Choose the Air Fry option on the Instant Pot Duo Crisp Air fryer. Set the temperature to 360°F and push start. The preheating will start.
2. Season your boneless turkey breast with mayonnaise, poultry seasoning, salt, garlic powder, and black pepper.
3. Once preheated, Air Fry the turkey breasts on 360°F for 1 hour, turning every 15 minutes or until internal temperature has reached a temperature of 165°F.

Nutrition Info: Calories 558, Total Fat 18g, Total Carbs 1g, Protein 98g

83. Air Fryer Fish

Servings: 4
Cooking Time: 17 Minutes
Ingredients:

- 4-6 Whiting Fish fillets cut in half
- Oil to mist
- Fish Seasoning
- ¾ cup very fine cornmeal
- ¼ cup flour
- 2 tsp old bay
- 1 ½ tsp salt
- 1 tsp paprika
- ½ tsp garlic powder
- ½ tsp black pepper

Directions:
1. Put the Ingredients: for fish seasoning in a Ziplock bag and shake it well. Set aside.
2. Rinse and pat dry the fish fillets with paper towels. Make sure that they still are damp.
3. Place the fish fillets in a ziplock bag and shake until they are completely covered with seasoning.
4. Place the fillets on a baking rack to let any excess flour to fall off.
5. Grease the bottom of the Instant Pot Duo Crisp Air Fryer basket tray and place the fillets on the tray. Close the lid, select the Air Fry option and cook filets on 400°F for 10 minutes.
6. Open the Air Fryer lid and spray the fish with oil on the side facing up before flipping it over, ensure that the fish is fully coated. Flip and cook another side of the fish for 7 minutes. Remove the fish and serve.

Nutrition Info: Calories 193, Total Fat 1g, Total Carbs 27g, Protein 19g

84. Chicken With Veggies And Rice

Servings: 3
Cooking Time: 20 Minutes
Ingredients:
- 3 cups cold boiled white rice
- 1 cup cooked chicken, diced
- ½ cup frozen carrots
- ½ cup frozen peas
- ½ cup onion, chopped
- 6 tablespoons soy sauce
- 1 tablespoon vegetable oil

Directions:
1. Preheat the Air fryer to 360 degree F and grease a 7" nonstick pan.
2. Mix the rice, soy sauce, and vegetable oil in a bowl.
3. Stir in the remaining ingredients and mix until well combined.
4. Transfer the rice mixture into the pan and place in the Air fryer.
5. Cook for about 20 minutes and dish out to serve immediately.

Nutrition Info: Calories: 405, Fat: 6.4g, Carbohydrates: 63g, Sugar: 3.5g, Protein: 21.7g, Sodium: 1500mg

85. Duck Breast With Figs

Servings: 2
Cooking Time: 45 Minutes
Ingredients:
- 1 pound boneless duck breast
- 6 fresh figs, halved
- 1 tablespoon fresh thyme, chopped
- 2 cups fresh pomegranate juice
- 2 tablespoons lemon juice
- 3 tablespoons brown sugar
- 1 teaspoon olive oil
- Salt and black pepper, as required

Directions:
1. Preheat the Air fryer to 400 degree F and grease an Air fryer basket.
2. Put the pomegranate juice, lemon juice, and brown sugar in a medium saucepan over medium heat.
3. Bring to a boil and simmer on low heat for about 25 minutes.
4. Season the duck breasts generously with salt and black pepper.
5. Arrange the duck breasts into the Air fryer basket, skin side up and cook for about 14 minutes, flipping once in between.
6. Dish out the duck breasts onto a cutting board for about 10 minutes.
7. Meanwhile, put the figs, olive oil, salt, and black pepper in a bowl until well mixed.
8. Set the Air fryer to 400 degree F and arrange the figs into the Air fryer basket.
9. Cook for about 5 more minutes and dish out in a platter.
10. Put the duck breast with the roasted figs and drizzle with warm pomegranate juice mixture.
11. Garnish with fresh thyme and serve warm.

Nutrition Info: Calories: 699, Fat: 12.1g, Carbohydrates: 90g, Sugar: 74g, Protein: 519g, Sodium: 110mg

86. Pecan Crunch Catfish And Asparagus

Servings: 4
Cooking Time: 12 Minutes
Ingredients:
- 1 cup whole wheat panko breadcrumbs
- 1/4 cup chopped pecans
- 3 teaspoons chopped fresh thyme
- 1-1/2 tablespoons extra-virgin olive oil, plus more for the pan

- Salt and pepper to taste
- 1-1/4 pounds asparagus
- 1 tablespoon honey
- 4 (5- to 6-ounce each) catfish filets

Directions:
1. Start by preheating toaster oven to 425°F.
2. Combine breadcrumbs, pecans, 2 teaspoons thyme, 1 tablespoon oil, salt, pepper and 2 tablespoons water.
3. In another bowl combine asparagus, the rest of the thyme, honey, salt, and pepper.
4. Spread the asparagus in a flat layer on a baking sheet. Sprinkle a quarter of the breadcrumb mixture over the asparagus.
5. Lay the catfish over the asparagus and press the rest of the breadcrumb mixture into each piece. Roast for 12 minutes.

Nutrition Info: Calories: 531, Sodium: 291 mg, Dietary Fiber: 6.1 g, Total Fat: 30.4 g, Total Carbs: 31.9 g, Protein: 34.8 g.

87. Roasted Garlic(2)

Servings: 12 Cloves
Cooking Time: 12 Minutes
Ingredients:
- 1 medium head garlic
- 2 tsp. avocado oil

Directions:
1. Remove any hanging excess peel from the garlic but leave the cloves covered. Cut off ¼ of the head of garlic, exposing the tips of the cloves
2. Drizzle with avocado oil. Place the garlic head into a small sheet of aluminum foil, completely enclosing it. Place it into the air fryer basket. Adjust the temperature to 400 Degrees F and set the timer for 20 minutes. If your garlic head is a bit smaller, check it after 15 minutes
3. When done, garlic should be golden brown and very soft
4. To serve, cloves should pop out and easily be spread or sliced. Store in an airtight container in the refrigerator up to 5 days.
5. You may also freeze individual cloves on a baking sheet, then store together in a freezer-safe storage bag once frozen.

Nutrition Info: Calories: 11; Protein: 2g; Fiber: 1g; Fat: 7g; Carbs: 0g

88. Beef Steaks With Beans

Servings: 4
Cooking Time: 10 Minutes
Ingredients:
- 4 beef steaks, trim the fat and cut into strips
- 1 cup green onions, chopped

- 2 cloves garlic, minced
- 1 red bell pepper, seeded and thinly sliced
- 1 can tomatoes, crushed
- 1 can cannellini beans
- 3/4 cup beef broth
- 1/4 teaspoon dried basil
- 1/2 teaspoon cayenne pepper
- 1/2 teaspoon sea salt
- 1/4 teaspoon ground black pepper, or to taste

Directions:
1. Preparing the ingredients. Add the steaks, green onions and garlic to the instant crisp air fryer basket.
2. Air frying. Close air fryer lid. Cook at 390 degrees f for 10 minutes, working in batches.
3. Stir in the remaining ingredients and cook for an additional 5 minutes.

Nutrition Info: Calories 284 Total fat 7.9 g Saturated fat 1.4 g Cholesterol 36 mg Sodium 704 mg Total carbs 46 g Fiber 3.6 g Sugar 5.5 g Protein 17.9 g

89. Zucchini And Cauliflower Stew

Servings: 4
Cooking Time: 12 Minutes
Ingredients:
- 1 cauliflower head, florets separated
- 1 ½ cups zucchinis; sliced
- 1 handful parsley leaves; chopped.
- ½ cup tomato puree
- 2 green onions; chopped.
- 1 tbsp. balsamic vinegar
- 1 tbsp. olive oil
- Salt and black pepper to taste.

Directions:
1. In a pan that fits your air fryer, mix the zucchinis with the rest of the ingredients except the parsley, toss, introduce the pan in the air fryer and cook at 380°F for 20 minutes
2. Divide into bowls and serve for lunch with parsley sprinkled on top.

Nutrition Info: Calories: 193; Fat: 5g; Fiber: 2g; Carbs: 4g; Protein: 7g

90. Chicken Potato Bake

Servings: 4
Cooking Time: 25 Minutes
Ingredients:
- 4 potatoes, diced
- 1 tablespoon garlic, minced
- 1.5 tablespoons olive oil
- 1/8 teaspoon salt
- 1/8 teaspoon pepper
- 1.5 lbs. boneless skinless chicken
- 3/4 cup mozzarella cheese, shredded

- parsley chopped

Directions:
1. Toss chicken and potatoes with all the spices and oil in a baking pan.
2. Drizzle the cheese on top of the chicken and potato.
3. Press "Power Button" of Air Fry Oven and turn the dial to select the "Bake" mode.
4. Press the Time button and again turn the dial to set the cooking time to 25 minutes.
5. Now push the Temp button and rotate the dial to set the temperature at 375 degrees F.
6. Once preheated, place the baking pan inside and close its lid.
7. Serve warm.

Nutrition Info: Calories 695 Total Fat 17.5 g Saturated Fat 4.8 g Cholesterol 283 mg Sodium 355 mg Total Carbs 26.4 g Fiber 1.8 g Sugar 0.8 g Protein 117.4 g

91. Marinated Chicken Parmesan

Servings: 4
Cooking Time: 20 Minutes
Ingredients:
- 2 cups breadcrumbs
- 1 teaspoon dried oregano
- 1/2 teaspoon garlic powder
- 4 teaspoons paprika
- 1/2 teaspoon salt
- 1/2 teaspoon black pepper
- 2 egg whites
- 1/2 cup skim milk
- 1/2 cup flour
- 4 (6 oz.) chicken breast halves, lb.ed
- Cooking spray
- 1 jar marinara sauce
- 3/4 cup mozzarella cheese, shredded
- 2 tablespoons Parmesan, shredded

Directions:
1. Whisk the flour with all the spices in a bowl and beat the eggs in another.
2. Coat the pounded chicken with flour then dip in the egg whites.
3. Dredge the chicken breast through the crumbs well.
4. Spread marinara sauce in a baking dish and place the crusted chicken on it.
5. Drizzle cheese on top of the chicken.
6. Press "Power Button" of Air Fry Oven and turn the dial to select the "Bake" mode.
7. Press the Time button and again turn the dial to set the cooking time to 20 minutes.
8. Now push the Temp button and rotate the dial to set the temperature at 400 degrees F.

9. Once preheated, place the baking pan inside and close its lid.
10. Serve warm.
Nutrition Info: Calories 361 Total Fat 16.3 g Saturated Fat 4.9 g Cholesterol 114 mg Sodium 515 mg Total Carbs 19.3 g Fiber 0.1 g Sugar 18.2 g Protein 33.3 g

92. Turkey Meatloaf

Servings: 4
Cooking Time: 20 Minutes
Ingredients:
- 1 pound ground turkey
- 1 cup kale leaves, trimmed and finely chopped
- 1 cup onion, chopped
- ½ cup fresh breadcrumbs
- 1 cup Monterey Jack cheese, grated
- 2 garlic cloves, minced
- ¼ cup salsa verde
- 1 teaspoon red chili powder
- ½ teaspoon ground cumin
- ½ teaspoon dried oregano, crushed
- Salt and ground black pepper, as required
Directions:
1. Preheat the Air fryer to 400 degree F and grease an Air fryer basket.
2. Mix all the ingredients in a bowl and divide the turkey mixture into 4 equal-sized portions.
3. Shape each into a mini loaf and arrange the loaves into the Air fryer basket.
4. Cook for about 20 minutes and dish out to serve warm.
Nutrition Info: Calories: 435, Fat: 23.1g, Carbohydrates: 18.1g, Sugar: 3.6g, Protein: 42.2g, Sodium: 641mg

93. Roasted Beet Salad With Oranges & Beet Greens

Servings: 6
Cooking Time: 1-1/2 Hours
Ingredients:
- 6 medium beets with beet greens attached
- 2 large oranges
- 1 small sweet onion, cut into wedges
- 1/3 cup red wine vinegar
- 1/4 cup extra-virgin olive oil
- 2 garlic cloves, minced
- 1/2 teaspoon grated orange peel
Directions:
1. Start by preheating toaster oven to 400°F.
2. Trim leaves from beets and chop, then set aside.
3. Pierce beets with a fork and place in a roasting pan.

4. Roast beets for 1-1/2 hours.
5. Allow beets to cool, peel, then cut into 8 wedges and put into a bowl.
6. Place beet greens in a sauce pan and cover with just enough water to cover. Heat until water boils, then immediately remove from heat.
7. Drain greens and press to remove liquid from greens, then add to beet bowl.
8. Remove peel and pith from orange and segment, adding each segment to the bowl.
9. Add onion to beet mixture. In a separate bowl mix together vinegar, oil, garlic and orange peel.
10. Combine both bowls and toss, sprinkle with salt and pepper.
11. Let stand for an hour before serving.
Nutrition Info: Calories: 214, Sodium: 183 mg, Dietary Fiber: 6.5 g, Total Fat: 8.9 g, Total Carbs: 32.4 g, Protein: 4.7 g.

94. Roasted Mini Peppers

Servings: 6
Cooking Time: 15 Minutes
Ingredients:
- 1 bag mini bell peppers
- Cooking spray
- Salt and pepper to taste
Directions:
1. Start by preheating toaster oven to 400°F.
2. Wash and dry the peppers, then place flat on a baking sheet.
3. Spray peppers with cooking spray and sprinkle with salt and pepper.
4. Roast for 15 minutes.
Nutrition Info: Calories: 19, Sodium: 2 mg, Dietary Fiber: 1.3 g, Total Fat: 0.3 g, Total Carbs: 3.6 g, Protein: 0.6 g.

95. Chicken And Celery Stew

Servings: 6
Cooking Time: 12 Minutes
Ingredients:
- 1 lb. chicken breasts, skinless; boneless and cubed
- 4 celery stalks; chopped.
- ½ cup coconut cream
- 2 red bell peppers; chopped.
- 2 tsp. garlic; minced
- 1 tbsp. butter, soft
- Salt and black pepper to taste.
Directions:
1. Grease a baking dish that fits your air fryer with the butter, add all the ingredients in the pan and toss them.

2. Introduce the dish in the fryer, cook at 360°F for 30 minutes, divide into bowls and serve
Nutrition Info: Calories: 246; Fat: 12g; Fiber: 2g; Carbs: 6g; Protein: 12g

96. Spanish Chicken Bake

Servings: 4
Cooking Time: 25 Minutes
Ingredients:
- ½ onion, quartered
- ½ red onion, quartered
- ½ lb. potatoes, quartered
- 4 garlic cloves
- 4 tomatoes, quartered
- 1/8 cup chorizo
- ¼ teaspoon paprika powder
- 4 chicken thighs, boneless
- ¼ teaspoon dried oregano
- ½ green bell pepper, julienned
- Salt
- Black pepper

Directions:
1. Toss chicken, veggies, and all the Ingredients: in a baking tray.
2. Press "Power Button" of Air Fry Oven and turn the dial to select the "Bake" mode.
3. Press the Time button and again turn the dial to set the cooking time to 25 minutes.
4. Now push the Temp button and rotate the dial to set the temperature at 425 degrees F.
5. Once preheated, place the baking pan inside and close its lid.
6. Serve warm.
Nutrition Info: Calories 301 Total Fat 8.9 g Saturated Fat 4.5 g Cholesterol 57 mg Sodium 340 mg Total Carbs 24.7 g Fiber 1.2 g Sugar 1.3 g Protein 15.3 g

97. Air Fried Sausages

Servings: 6
Cooking Time: 13 Minutes
Ingredients:
- 6 sausage
- olive oil spray

Directions:
1. Pour 5 cup of water into Instant Pot Duo Crisp Air Fryer. Place air fryer basket inside the pot, spray inside with nonstick spray and put sausage links inside.
2. Close the Air Fryer lid and steam for about 5 minutes.
3. Remove the lid once done. Spray links with olive oil and close air crisp lid.

4. Set to air crisp at 400°F for 8 min flipping halfway through so both sides get browned.
Nutrition Info: Calories 267, Total Fat 23g, Total Carbs 2g, Protein 13g

98. Crispy Breaded Pork Chop

Servings: 6
Cooking Time: 12 Minutes
Ingredients:
- olive oil spray
- 6 3/4-inch thick center-cut boneless pork chops, fat trimmed (5 oz each)
- kosher salt
- 1 large egg, beaten
- 1/2 cup panko crumbs, check labels for GF
- 1/3 cup crushed cornflakes crumbs
- 2 tbsp grated parmesan cheese
- 1 1/4 tsp sweet paprika
- 1/2 tsp garlic powder
- 1/2 tsp onion powder
- 1/4 tsp chili powder
- 1/8 tsp black pepper

Directions:
1. Preheat the Instant Pot Duo Crisp Air Fryer for 12 minutes at 400°F.
2. On both sides, season pork chops with half teaspoon kosher salt.
3. Then combine cornflake crumbs, panko, parmesan cheese, 3/4 tsp kosher salt, garlic powder, paprika, onion powder, chili powder, and black pepper in a large bowl.
4. Place the egg beat in another bowl. Dip the pork in the egg & then crumb mixture.
5. When the air fryer is ready, place 3 of the chops into the Instant Pot Duo Crisp Air Fryer Basket and spritz the top with oil.
6. Close the Air Fryer lid and cook for 12 minutes turning halfway, spritzing both sides with oil.
7. Set aside and repeat with the remaining.
Nutrition Info: Calories 281, Total Fat 13g, Total Carbs 8g, Protein 33g

99. Vegetarian Philly Sandwich

Servings: 2
Cooking Time: 20 Minutes
Ingredients:
- 2 tablespoons olive oil
- 8 ounces sliced portabello mushrooms
- 1 vidalia onion, thinly sliced
- 1 green bell pepper, thinly sliced
- 1 red bell pepper, thinly sliced
- Salt and pepper
- 4 slices 2% provolone cheese

- 4 rolls

Directions:
1. Preheat toaster oven to 475°F.
2. Heat the oil in a medium sauce pan over medium heat.
3. Sauté mushrooms about 5 minutes, then add the onions and peppers and sauté another 10 minutes.
4. Slice rolls lengthwise and divide the vegetables into each roll.
5. Add the cheese and toast until the rolls start to brown and the cheese melts.

Nutrition Info: Calories: 645, Sodium: 916 mg, Dietary Fiber: 7.2 g, Total Fat: 33.3 g, Total Carbs: 61.8 g, Protein: 27.1 g.

100.Jicama Fries(1)

Servings: 4
Cooking Time: 12 Minutes
Ingredients:
- 1 small jicama; peeled.
- ¼ tsp. onion powder.
- ¾tsp. chili powder
- ¼ tsp. ground black pepper
- ¼ tsp. garlic powder.

Directions:
1. Cut jicama into matchstick-sized pieces.
2. Place pieces into a small bowl and sprinkle with remaining ingredients. Place the fries into the air fryer basket
3. Adjust the temperature to 350 Degrees F and set the timer for 20 minutes. Toss the basket two or three times during cooking. Serve warm.

Nutrition Info: Calories: 37; Protein: 8g; Fiber: 7g; Fat: 1g; Carbs: 7g

101.Sweet Potato Rosti

Servings: 2
Cooking Time: 15 Minutes
Ingredients:
- ½ lb. sweet potatoes, peeled, grated and squeezed
- 1 tablespoon fresh parsley, chopped finely
- Salt and ground black pepper, as required
- 2 tablespoons sour cream

Directions:
1. In a large bowl, mix together the grated sweet potato, parsley, salt, and black pepper.
2. Press "Power Button" of Air Fry Oven and turn the dial to select the "Air Fry" mode.
3. Press the Time button and again turn the dial to set the cooking time to 15 minutes.
4. Now push the Temp button and rotate the dial to set the temperature at 355 degrees F.

5. Press "Start/Pause" button to start.
6. When the unit beeps to show that it is preheated, open the lid and lightly, grease the sheet pan.
7. Arrange the sweet potato mixture into the "Sheet Pan" and shape it into an even circle.
8. Insert the "Sheet Pan" in the oven.
9. Cut the potato rosti into wedges.
10. Top with the sour cream and serve immediately.

Nutrition Info: Calories: 160 Cal Total Fat: 2.7 g Saturated Fat: 1.6 g Cholesterol: 5 mg Sodium: 95 mg Total Carbs: 32.3 g Fiber: 4.7 g Sugar: 0.6 g Protein: 2.2 g

102.Spice-roasted Almonds

Servings: 32
Cooking Time: 10 Minutes
Ingredients:
- 1 tablespoon chili powder
- 1 tablespoon olive oil
- 1/2 teaspoon salt
- 1/2 teaspoon ground cumin
- 1/2 teaspoon ground coriander
- 1/4 teaspoon ground cinnamon
- 1/4 teaspoon black pepper
- 2 cups whole almonds

Directions:
1. Start by preheating toaster oven to 350°F.
2. Mix olive oil, chili powder, coriander, cinnamon, cumin, salt, and pepper.
3. Add almonds and toss together.
4. Transfer to a baking pan and bake for 10 minutes.

Nutrition Info: Calories: 39, Sodium: 37 mg, Dietary Fiber: 0.8 g, Total Fat: 3.5 g, Total Carbs: 1.4 g, Protein: 1.3 g.

103.Kalamta Mozarella Pita Melts

Servings: 2
Cooking Time: 5 Minutes
Ingredients:
- 2 (6-inch) whole wheat pitas
- 1 teaspoon extra-virgin olive oil
- 1 cup grated part-skim mozzarella cheese
- 1/4 small red onion
- 1/4 cup pitted Kalamata olives
- 2 tablespoons chopped fresh herbs such as parsley, basil, or oregano

Directions:
1. Start by preheating toaster oven to 425°F.
2. Brush the pita on both sides with oil and warm in the oven for one minute.
3. Dice onions and halve olives.

4. Sprinkle mozzarella over each pita and top with onion and olive.
5. Return to the oven for another 5 minutes or until the cheese is melted.
6. Sprinkle herbs over the pita and serve.
Nutrition Info: Calories: 387, Sodium: 828 mg, Dietary Fiber: 7.4 g, Total Fat: 16.2 g, Total Carbs: 42.0 g, Protein: 23.0 g.

104. Delicious Chicken Burgers

Servings: 4
Cooking Time: 30 Minutes
Ingredients:
- 4 boneless, skinless chicken breasts
- 1¾ ounces plain flour
- 2 eggs
- 4 hamburger buns, split and toasted
- 4 mozzarella cheese slices
- 1 teaspoon mustard powder
- ½ teaspoon paprika
- 1 teaspoon Worcestershire sauce
- ¼ teaspoon dried parsley
- ¼ teaspoon dried tarragon
- ¼ teaspoon dried oregano
- 1 teaspoon dried garlic
- 1 teaspoon chicken seasoning
- ½ teaspoon cayenne pepper
- Salt and black pepper, as required

Directions:
1. Preheat the Air fryer to 355 degree F and grease an Air fryer basket.
2. Put the chicken breasts, mustard, paprika, Worcestershire sauce, salt, and black pepper in a food processor and pulse until minced.
3. Make 4 equal-sized patties from the mixture.
4. Place the flour in a shallow bowl and whisk the egg in a second bowl.
5. Combine dried herbs and spices in a third bowl.
6. Coat each chicken patty with flour, dip into whisked egg and then coat with breadcrumb mixture.
7. Arrange the chicken patties into the Air fryer basket in a single layer and cook for about 30 minutes, flipping once in between.
8. Place half bun in a plate, layer with lettuce leaf, patty and cheese slice.
9. Cover with bun top and dish out to serve warm.
Nutrition Info: Calories: 562, Fat: 20.3g, Carbohydrates: 33g, Sugar: 3.3g, Protein: 58.7g, Sodium: 560mg

105. Chicken Breast With Rosemary

Servings: 4
Cooking Time: 60 Minutes

Ingredients:
- 4 bone-in chicken breast halves
- 3 tablespoons softened butter
- 1/2 teaspoon salt
- 1/4 teaspoon pepper
- 1 tablespoon rosemary
- 1 tablespoon extra-virgin olive oil

Directions:
1. Start by preheating toaster oven to 400°F.
2. Mix butter, salt, pepper, and rosemary in a bowl.
3. Coat chicken with the butter mixture and place in a shallow pan.
4. Drizzle oil over chicken and roast for 25 minutes.
5. Flip chicken and roast for another 20 minutes.
6. Flip chicken one more time and roast for a final 15 minutes.
Nutrition Info: Calories: 392, Sodium: 551 mg, Dietary Fiber: 0 g, Total Fat: 18.4 g, Total Carbs: 0.6 g, Protein: 55.4 g.

106. Sweet Potato Chips

Servings: 2
Cooking Time: 40 Minutes
Ingredients:
- 2 sweet potatoes
- Salt and pepper to taste
- Olive oil
- Cinnamon

Directions:
1. Start by preheating toaster oven to 400°F.
2. Cut off each end of potato and discard.
3. Cut potatoes into 1/2-inch slices.
4. Brush a pan with olive oil and lay potato slices flat on the pan.
5. Bake for 20 minutes, then flip and bake for another 20.
Nutrition Info: Calories: 139, Sodium: 29 mg, Dietary Fiber: 8.2 g, Total Fat: 0.5 g, Total Carbs: 34.1 g, Protein: 1.9 g.

107. Air Fryer Marinated Salmon

Servings: 4
Cooking Time: 12 Minutes
Ingredients:
- 4 salmon fillets or 1 1lb fillet cut into 4 pieces
- 1 Tbsp brown sugar
- ½ Tbsp Minced Garlic
- 6 Tbsps Soy Sauce
- ¼ cup Dijon Mustard
- 1 Green onions finely chopped

Directions:
1. Take a bowl and whisk together soy sauce, dijon mustard, brown sugar, and minced garlic. Pour this mixture over salmon fillets, making sure that all the

fillets are covered. Refrigerate and marinate for 20-30 minutes.

2. Remove salmon fillets from marinade and place them in greased or lined on the tray in the Instant Pot Duo Crisp Air Fryer basket, close the lid.

3. Select the Air Fry option and Air Fry for around 12 minutes at 400°F.

4. Remove from Instant Pot Duo Crisp Air Fryer and top with chopped green onions.

Nutrition Info: Calories 267, Total Fat 11g, Total Carbs 5g, Protein 37g

108.Easy Italian Meatballs

Servings: 4
Cooking Time: 13 Minutes
Ingredients:
- 2-lb. lean ground turkey
- ¼ cup onion, minced
- 2 cloves garlic, minced
- 2 tablespoons parsley, chopped
- 2 eggs
- 1½ cup parmesan cheese, grated
- ½ teaspoon red pepper flakes
- ½ teaspoon Italian seasoning Salt and black pepper to taste

Directions:
1. Toss all the meatball Ingredients: in a bowl and mix well.
2. Make small meatballs out this mixture and place them in the air fryer basket.
3. Press "Power Button" of Air Fry Oven and turn the dial to select the "Air Fry" mode.
4. Press the Time button and again turn the dial to set the cooking time to 13 minutes.
5. Now push the Temp button and rotate the dial to set the temperature at 350 degrees F.
6. Once preheated, place the air fryer basket inside and close its lid.
7. Flip the meatballs when cooked halfway through.
8. Serve warm.

Nutrition Info: Calories 472 Total Fat 25.8 g Saturated Fat .4 g Cholesterol 268 mg Sodium 503 mg Total Carbs 1.7 g Fiber 0.3 g Sugar 0.6 g Protein 59.6 g

109.Mushroom Meatloaf

Servings: 4
Cooking Time: 25 Minutes
Ingredients:
- 14-ounce lean ground beef
- 1 chorizo sausage, chopped finely
- 1 small onion, chopped
- 1 garlic clove, minced
- 2 tablespoons fresh cilantro, chopped
- 3 tablespoons breadcrumbs
- 1 egg
- Salt and freshly ground black pepper, to taste

- 2 tablespoons fresh mushrooms, sliced thinly
- 3 tablespoons olive oil

Directions:
1. Preparing the ingredients. Preheat the instant crisp air fryer to 390 degrees f.
2. In a large bowl, add all ingredients except mushrooms and mix till well combined.
3. In a baking pan, place the beef mixture.
4. With the back of spatula, smooth the surface.
5. Top with mushroom slices and gently, press into the meatloaf.
6. Drizzle with oil evenly.
7. Air frying. Arrange the pan in the instant crisp air fryer basket, close air fryer lid and cook for about 25 minutes.
8. Cut the meatloaf in desires size wedges and serve.

Nutrition Info: Calories 284 Total fat 7.9 g Saturated fat 1.4 g Cholesterol 36 mg Sodium 704 mg Total carbs 46 g Fiber 3.6 g Sugar 5.5 g Protein 17.9 g

110.Lime And Mustard Marinated Chicken

Servings: 4
Cooking Time: 10 Minutes
Ingredients:
- 1/2 teaspoon stone-ground mustard
- 1/2 teaspoon minced fresh oregano
- 1/3 cup freshly squeezed lime juice
- 2 small-sized chicken breasts, skin-on
- 1 teaspoon kosher salt
- 1teaspoon freshly cracked mixed peppercorns

Directions:
1. Preheat your Air Fryer to 345 degrees F.
2. Toss all of the above ingredients in a medium-sized mixing dish; allow it to marinate overnight.
3. Cook in the preheated Air Fryer for 26 minutes.

Nutrition Info: 255 Calories; 15g Fat; 7g Carbs; 33g Protein; 8g Sugars; 3g Fiber

111.Seven-layer Tostadas

Servings: 6
Cooking Time: 5 Minutes
Ingredients:
- 1 (16-ounce) can refried pinto beans
- 1-1/2 cups guacamole
- 1 cup light sour cream
- 1/2 teaspoon taco seasoning
- 1 cup shredded Mexican cheese blend
- 1 cup chopped tomatoes
- 1/2 cup thinly sliced green onions
- 1/2 cup sliced black olives
- 6-8 whole wheat flour tortillas small enough to fit in your oven
- Olive oil

Directions:

1. Start by placing baking sheet into toaster oven while preheating it to 450°F. Remove pan and drizzle with olive oil.
2. Place tortillas on pan and cook in oven until they are crisp, turn at least once, this should take about 5 minutes or less.
3. In a medium bowl, mash refried beans to break apart any chunks, then microwave for 2 1/2 minutes.
4. Stir taco seasoning into the sour cream. Chop vegetables and halve olives.
5. Top tortillas with ingredients in this order: refried beans, guacamole, sour cream, shredded cheese, tomatoes, onions, and olives.
Nutrition Info: Calories: 657, Sodium: 581 mg, Dietary Fiber: 16.8 g, Total Fat: 31.7 g, Total Carbs: 71.3 g, Protein: 28.9 g.

112. Turkey And Broccoli Stew

Servings: 4
Cooking Time: 12 Minutes
Ingredients:
- 1 broccoli head, florets separated
- 1 turkey breast, skinless; boneless and cubed
- 1 cup tomato sauce
- 1 tbsp. parsley; chopped.
- 1 tbsp. olive oil
- Salt and black pepper to taste.

Directions:
1. In a baking dish that fits your air fryer, mix the turkey with the rest of the ingredients except the parsley, toss, introduce the dish in the fryer, bake at 380°F for 25 minutes
2. Divide into bowls, sprinkle the parsley on top and serve.
Nutrition Info: Calories: 250; Fat: 11g; Fiber: 2g; Carbs: 6g; Protein: 12g

113. Lobster Tails

Servings: 2
Cooking Time: 8 Minutes
Ingredients:
- 2 6oz lobster tails
- 1 tsp salt
- 1 tsp chopped chives
- 2 Tbsp unsalted butter melted
- 1 Tbsp minced garlic
- 1 tsp lemon juice

Directions:

1. Combine butter, garlic, salt, chives, and lemon juice to prepare butter mixture.
2. Butterfly lobster tails by cutting through shell followed by removing the meat and resting it on top of the shell.
3. Place them on the tray in the Instant Pot Duo Crisp Air Fryer basket and spread butter over the top of lobster meat. Close the Air Fryer lid, select the Air Fry option and cook on 380°F for 4 minutes.
4. Open the Air Fryer lid and spread more butter on top, cook for extra 2-4 minutes until done.
Nutrition Info: Calories 120, Total Fat 12g, Total Carbs 2g, Protein 1g

114. Sweet Potato And Parsnip Spiralized Latkes

Servings: 12
Cooking Time: 20 Minutes
Ingredients:
- 1 medium sweet potato
- 1 large parsnip
- 4 cups water
- 1 egg + 1 egg white
- 2 scallions
- 1/2 teaspoon garlic powder
- 1/2 teaspoon sea salt
- 1/2 teaspoon ground pepper

Directions:
1. Start by spiralizing the sweet potato and parsnip and chopping the scallions, reserving only the green parts.
2. Preheat toaster oven to 425°F.
3. Bring 4 cups of water to a boil. Place all of your noodles in a colander and pour the boiling water over the top, draining well.
4. Let the noodles cool, then grab handfuls and place them in a paper towel; squeeze to remove as much liquid as possible.
5. In a large bowl, beat egg and egg white together. Add noodles, scallions, garlic powder, salt, and pepper, mix well.
6. Prepare a baking sheet; scoop out 1/4 cup of mixture at a time and place on sheet.
7. Slightly press down each scoop with your hands, then bake for 20 minutes, flipping halfway through.
Nutrition Info: Calories: 24, Sodium: 91 mg, Dietary Fiber: 1.0 g, Total Fat: 0.4 g, Total Carbs: 4.3 g, Protein: 0.9 g.

DINNER RECIPES

115. Curried Eggplant

Servings: 2
Cooking Time: 10 Minutes
Ingredients:
- 1 large eggplant, cut into ½-inch thick slices
- 1 garlic clove, minced
- ½ fresh red chili, chopped
- 1 tablespoon vegetable oil
- ¼ teaspoon curry powder
- Salt, to taste

Directions:
1. Preheat the Air fryer to 300 degree F and grease an Air fryer basket.
2. Mix all the ingredients in a bowl and toss to coat well.
3. Arrange the eggplant slices in the Air fryer basket and cook for about 10 minutes, tossing once in between.
4. Dish out onto serving plates and serve hot.
Nutrition Info: Calories: 121, Fat: 7.3g, Carbohydrates: 14.2g, Sugar: 7g, Protein: 2.4g, Sodium: 83mg

116. Adobe Turkey Chimichangas

Servings: 4
Cooking Time: 15 Minutes
Ingredients:
- 1 pound thickly-sliced smoked turkey from deli counter, chopped
- 1 tablespoon chili powder
- 2 cups shredded slaw cabbage
- 1 to 2 chipotles in adobo sauce
- 1 cup tomato sauce
- 3 chopped scallions
- Salt and pepper
- 4 (12-inch) flour tortillas
- 1-1/2 cups pepper jack cheese
- 2 tablespoons olive oil
- 1 cup sour cream
- 2 tablespoons chopped cilantro

Directions:
1. Start by preheating toaster oven to 400°F.
2. In a medium bowl mix together turkey and chili powder.
3. Add cabbage, chipotles, tomato sauce, and scallions; mix well.
4. Season cabbage mixture with salt and pepper and turn a few times.
5. Warm tortillas in a microwave or on a stove top.
6. Lay cheese flat in each tortilla and top with turkey mixture.

7. Fold in the top and bottom of the tortilla, then roll to close.
8. Brush baking tray with oil, then place chimichangas on tray and brush with oil.
9. Bake for 15 minutes or until tortilla is golden brown.
10. Top with sour cream and cilantro and serve.
Nutrition Info: Calories: 638, Sodium: 1785 mg, Dietary Fiber: 4.2 g, Total Fat: 44.0 g, Total Carbs: 23.9 g, Protein: 38.4 g.

117. Sweet Chicken Breast

Servings: 4
Cooking Time: 12 Minutes
Ingredients:
- 1-pound chicken breast, boneless, skinless
- 3 tablespoon Stevia extract
- 1 teaspoon ground white pepper
- ½ teaspoon paprika
- 1 teaspoon cayenne pepper
- 1 teaspoon lemongrass
- 1 teaspoon lemon zest
- 1 tablespoon apple cider vinegar
- 1 tablespoon butter

Directions:
1. Sprinkle the chicken breast with the apple cider vinegar.
2. After this, rub the chicken breast with the ground white pepper, paprika, cayenne pepper, lemongrass, and lemon zest.
3. Leave the chicken breast for 5 minutes to marinate.
4. After this, rub the chicken breast with the stevia extract and leave it for 5 minutes more.
5. Preheat the air fryer to 380 F.
6. Rub the prepared chicken breast with the butter and place it in the air fryer basket tray.
7. Cook the chicken breast for 12 minutes.
8. Turn the chicken breast into another side after 6 minutes of cooking.
9. Serve the dish hot!
10. Enjoy!
Nutrition Info: calories 160, fat 5.9, fiber 0.4, carbs 1, protein 24.2

118. Easy Marinated London Broil

Servings: 4
Cooking Time: 20 Minutes
Ingredients:
- For the marinade:
- 2 tablespoons Worcestershire sauce
- 2 garlic cloves, minced

- 1 tablespoon oil
- 2 tablespoons rice vinegar
- London Broil:
- 2 pounds London broil
- 2 tablespoons tomato paste
- Sea salt and cracked black pepper, to taste
- 1 tablespoon mustard

Directions:
1. Combine all the marinade ingredients in a mixing bowl; add the London boil to the bowl. Cover and let it marinate for 3 hours.
2. Preheat the Air Fryer to 400 degrees F. Spritz the Air Fryer grill pan with cooking oil.
3. Grill the marinated London broil in the preheated Air Fryer for 18 minutes. Turn London broil over, top with the tomato paste, salt, black pepper, and mustard.
4. Continue to grill an additional 10 minutes. Serve immediately.

Nutrition Info: 517 Calories; 21g Fat; 5g Carbs; 70g Protein; 4g Sugars; 7g Fiber

119.Coconut Crusted Shrimp

Servings: 3
Cooking Time: 40 Minutes
Ingredients:
- 8 ounces coconut milk
- ½ cup sweetened coconut, shredded
- ½ cup panko breadcrumbs
- 1 pound large shrimp, peeled and deveined
- Salt and black pepper, to taste

Directions:
1. Preheat the Air fryer to 350-degree F and grease an Air fryer basket.
2. Place the coconut milk in a shallow bowl.
3. Mix coconut, breadcrumbs, salt, and black pepper in another bowl.
4. Dip each shrimp into coconut milk and finally, dredge in the coconut mixture.
5. Arrange half of the shrimps into the Air fryer basket and cook for about 20 minutes.
6. Dish out the shrimps onto serving plates and repeat with the remaining mixture to serve.

Nutrition Info: Calories: 408, Fats: 23.7g, Carbohydrates: 11.7g, Sugar: 3.4g, Proteins: 31g, Sodium: 253mg

120.Green Beans And Mushroom Casserole

Servings: 6
Cooking Time: 12 Minutes
Ingredients:
- 24 ounces fresh green beans, trimmed

- 2 cups fresh button mushrooms, sliced
- 1/3 cup French fried onions
- 3 tablespoons olive oil
- 2 tablespoons fresh lemon juice
- 1 teaspoon ground sage
- 1 teaspoon garlic powder
- 1 teaspoon onion powder
- Salt and black pepper, to taste

Directions:
1. Preheat the Air fryer to 400F and grease an Air fryer basket.
2. Mix the green beans, mushrooms, oil, lemon juice, sage, and spices in a bowl and toss to coat well.
3. Arrange the green beans mixture into the Air fryer basket and cook for about 12 minutes.
4. Dish out in a serving dish and top with fried onions to serve.

Nutrition Info: Calories: 65, Fat: 1.6g, Carbohydrates: 11g, Sugar: 2.4g, Protein: 3g, Sodium: 52mg

121.Garlic Butter Pork Chops

Servings: 4
Cooking Time: 8 Minutes
Ingredients:
- 4 pork chops
- 1 tablespoon coconut butter
- 2 teaspoons parsley
- 1 tablespoon coconut oil
- 2 teaspoons garlic, grated
- Salt and black pepper, to taste

Directions:
1. Preheat the Air fryer to 350 degree F and grease an Air fryer basket.
2. Mix all the seasonings, coconut oil, garlic, butter, and parsley in a bowl and coat the pork chops with it.
3. Cover the chops with foil and refrigerate to marinate for about 1 hour.
4. Remove the foil and arrange the chops in the Air fryer basket.
5. Cook for about 8 minutes and dish out in a bowl to serve warm.

Nutrition Info: Calories: 311, Fat: 25.5g, Carbohydrates: 1.4g, Sugar: 0.3g, Protein: 18.4g, Sodium: 58mg

122.Beef, Mushrooms And Noodles Dish

Servings: 5
Cooking Time: 35 Minutes
Ingredients:
- 1½ pounds beef steak
- 1 package egg noodles, cooked
- 1 ounce dry onion soup mix
- 1 can (15 oz cream mushroom soup

- 2 cups mushrooms, sliced
- 1 whole onion, chopped
- ½ cup beef broth
- 3 garlic cloves, minced?

Directions:

1. Preheat your Air Fryer to 360 F. Drizzle onion soup mix all over the meat. In a mixing bowl, mix the sauce, garlic cloves, beef broth, chopped onion, sliced mushrooms and mushroom soup. Top the meat with the prepared sauce mixture. Place the prepared meat in the air fryer's cooking basket and cook for 25 minutes. Serve with cooked egg noodles.

Nutrition Info: 346 Calories; 11g Fat; 4g Carbs; 32g Protein; 1g Sugars; 1g Fiber

123.Zucchini Muffins

Servings: 8
Cooking Time: 20 Minutes
Ingredients:

- 6 eggs
- 4 drops stevia 1/4 cup Swerve
- 1/3 cup coconut oil, melted 1 cup zucchini, grated
- 3/4 cup coconut flour 1/4 tsp ground nutmeg 1 tsp ground cinnamon 1/2 tsp baking soda

Directions:

1. Preheat the air fryer to 325 F.
2. Add all ingredients except zucchini in a bowl and mix well.
3. Add zucchini and stir well.
4. Pour batter into the silicone muffin molds and place into the air fryer basket.
5. Cook muffins for 20 minutes.
6. Serve and enjoy.

Nutrition Info: Calories 136 Fat 12 g Carbohydrates 1 g Sugar 0.6 g Protein 4 g Cholesterol 123 mg

124.Cheddar Pork Meatballs

Servings: 4 To 6
Cooking Time: 25 Minutes
Ingredients:

- 1 lb ground pork
- 1 large onion, chopped
- ½ tsp maple syrup
- 2 tsp mustard
- ½ cup chopped basil leaves
- Salt and black pepper to taste
- 2 tbsp. grated cheddar cheese

Directions:

1. In a mixing bowl, add the ground pork, onion, maple syrup, mustard, basil leaves, salt, pepper, and cheddar cheese; mix well. Use your hands to form

bite-size balls. Place in the fryer basket and cook at 400 f for 10 minutes.

2. Slide out the fryer basket and shake it to toss the meatballs. Cook further for 5 minutes. Remove them onto a wire rack and serve with zoodles and marinara sauce.

Nutrition Info: Calories: 300 Cal Total Fat: 24 g Saturated Fat: 9 g Cholesterol: 70 mg Sodium: 860 mg Total Carbs: 3 g Fiber: 0 g Sugar: 0 g Protein: 16 g

125.Cinnamon Pork Rinds

Servings: 2
Cooking Time: 20 Minutes
Ingredients:

- 2 oz. pork rinds
- ¼ cup powdered erythritol
- 2 tbsp. unsalted butter; melted.
- ½ tsp. ground cinnamon.

Directions:

1. Take a large bowl, toss pork rinds and butter. Sprinkle with cinnamon and erythritol, then toss to evenly coat.
2. Place pork rinds into the air fryer basket. Adjust the temperature to 400 Degrees F and set the timer for 5 minutes. Serve immediately.

Nutrition Info: Calories: 264; Protein: 13g; Fiber: 4g; Fat: 28g; Carbs: 15g

126.Hasselback Potatoes

Servings: 4
Cooking Time: 30 Minutes
Ingredients:

- 4 potatoes
- 2 tablespoons Parmesan cheese, shredded
- 1 tablespoon fresh chives, chopped
- 2 tablespoons olive oil

Directions:

1. Preheat the Air fryer to 355F and grease an Air fryer basket.
2. Cut slits along each potato about ¼-inch apart with a sharp knife, making sure slices should stay connected at the bottom.
3. Coat the potatoes with olive oil and arrange into the Air fryer basket.
4. Cook for about 30 minutes and dish out in a platter.
5. Top with chives and Parmesan cheese to serve.

Nutrition Info: Calories: 218, Fat: 7.9g, Carbohydrates: 33.6g, Sugar: 2.5g, Protein: 4.6g, Sodium: 55mg

127.Baby Portabellas With Romano Cheese

Servings: 4
Cooking Time: 20 Minutes
Ingredients:
- 1 pound baby portabellas
- 1/2 cup almond meal
- 2 eggs
- 2 tablespoons milk
- 1 cup Romano cheese, grated
- Sea salt and ground black pepper
- 1/2 teaspoon shallot powder
- 1 teaspoon garlic powder
- 1/2 teaspoon cumin powder
- 1/2 teaspoon cayenne pepper

Directions:
1. Pat the mushrooms dry with a paper towel.
2. To begin, set up your breading station. Place the almond meal in a shallow dish. In a separate dish, whisk the eggs with milk.
3. Finally, place grated Romano cheese and seasonings in the third dish.
4. Start by dredging the baby portabellas in the almond meal mixture; then, dip them into the egg wash. Press the baby portabellas into Romano cheese, coating evenly.
5. Spritz the Air Fryer basket with cooking oil. Add the baby portabellas and cook at 400 degrees F for 6 minutes, flipping them halfway through the cooking time.

Nutrition Info: 230 Calories; 13g Fat; 2g Carbs; 11g Protein; 8g Sugars; 6g Fiber

128.Grilled Chicken Tikka Masala

Servings: 4
Cooking Time: 20 Minutes
Ingredients:
- 1 tsp. Tikka Masala 1 tsp. fine sea salt
- 2 heaping tsps. whole grain mustard
- 2 tsps. coriander, ground 2 tablespoon olive oil
- 2 large-sized chicken breasts, skinless and halved lengthwise
- 2 tsp.s onion powder
- 1½ tablespoons cider vinegar Basmati rice, steamed
- 1/3 tsp. red pepper flakes, crushed

Directions:
1. Preheat the air fryer to 335 °For 4 minutes.
2. Toss your chicken together with the other ingredients, minus basmati rice. Let it stand at least 3 hours.
3. Cook for 25 minutes in your air fryer; check for doneness because the time depending on the size of the piece of chicken.

4. Serve immediately over warm basmati rice. Enjoy!
Nutrition Info: 319 Calories; 20.1g Fat; 1.9g Carbs; 30.5g Protein; 0.1g Sugars

129.Kale And Brussels Sprouts

Servings: 8
Cooking Time: 7 Minutes
Ingredients:
- 1 lb. Brussels sprouts, trimmed
- 3 oz. mozzarella, shredded
- 2 cups kale, torn
- 1 tbsp. olive oil
- Salt and black pepper to taste.

Directions:
1. In a pan that fits the air fryer, combine all the Ingredients: except the mozzarella and toss.
2. Put the pan in the air fryer and cook at 380°F for 15 minutes
3. Divide between plates, sprinkle the cheese on top and serve.
Nutrition Info: Calories: 170; Fat: 5g; Fiber: 3g; Carbs: 4g; Protein: 7g

130.Miso-glazed Salmon

Servings: 4
Cooking Time: 5 Minutes
Ingredients:
- 1/4 cup red or white miso
- 1/3 cup sake
- 1 tablespoon soy sauce
- 2 tablespoons vegetable oil
- 1/4 cup sugar
- 4 skinless salmon filets

Directions:
1. In a shallow bowl, mix together the miso, sake, oil, soy sauce, and sugar.
2. Toss the salmon in the mixture until thoroughly coated on all sides.
3. Preheat your toaster oven to "high" on broil mode.
4. Place salmon in a broiling pan and broil until the top is well charred—about 5 minutes.
Nutrition Info: Calories: 401, Sodium: 315 mg, Dietary Fiber: 0 g, Total Fat: 19.2 g, Total Carbs: 14.1 g, Protein: 39.2 g.

131.Bbq Pork Ribs

Servings: 2 To 3
Cooking Time: 5 Hrs 30 Minutes
Ingredients:
- 1 lb pork ribs

- 1 tsp soy sauce
- Salt and black pepper to taste
- 1 tsp oregano
- 1 tbsp + 1 tbsp maple syrup
- 3 tbsp barbecue sauce
- 2 cloves garlic, minced
- 1 tbsp cayenne pepper
- 1 tsp sesame oil

Directions:

1. Put the chops on a chopping board and use a knife to cut them into smaller pieces of desired sizes. Put them in a mixing bowl, add the soy sauce, salt, pepper, oregano, one tablespoon of maple syrup, barbecue sauce, garlic, cayenne pepper, and sesame oil. Mix well and place the pork in the fridge to marinate in the spices for 5 hours.
2. Preheat the Air Fryer to 350 F. Open the Air Fryer and place the ribs in the fryer basket. Slide the fryer basket in and cook for 15 minutes. Open the Air fryer, turn the ribs using tongs, apply the remaining maple syrup with a brush, close the Air Fryer, and continue cooking for 10 minutes.

Nutrition Info: 346 Calories; 11g Fat; 4g Carbs; 32g Protein; 1g Sugars; 1g Fiber

132.Rich Meatloaf With Mustard And Peppers

Servings: 5
Cooking Time: 20 Minutes
Ingredients:

- 1 pound beef, ground
- 1/2 pound veal, ground
- 1 egg
- 4 tablespoons vegetable juice
- 1/2 cup pork rinds
- 2 bell peppers, chopped
- 1 onion, chopped
- 2 garlic cloves, minced
- 2 tablespoons tomato paste
- 2 tablespoons soy sauce
- 1 (1-ouncepackage ranch dressing mix
- Sea salt, to taste
- 1/2 teaspoon ground black pepper, to taste
- 7 ounces tomato puree
- 1 tablespoon Dijon mustard

Directions:

1. Start by preheating your Air Fryer to 330 degrees F.
2. In a mixing bowl, thoroughly combine the ground beef, veal, egg, vegetable juice, pork rinds, bell peppers, onion, garlic, tomato paste, soy sauce, ranch dressing mix, salt, and ground black pepper.
3. Mix until everything is well incorporated and press into a lightly greased meatloaf pan.

4. Cook approximately 25 minutes in the preheated Air Fryer. Whisk the tomato puree with the mustard and spread the topping over the top of your meatloaf.
5. Continue to cook 2 minutes more. Let it stand on a cooling rack for 6 minutes before slicing and serving. Enjoy!

Nutrition Info: 398 Calories; 24g Fat; 9g Carbs; 32g Protein; 3g Sugars; 6g Fiber

133.Basil Tomatoes

Servings: 2
Cooking Time: 10 Minutes
Ingredients:

- 2 tomatoes, halved
- 1 tablespoon fresh basil, chopped
- Olive oil cooking spray
- Salt and black pepper, as required

Directions:

1. Preheat the Air fryer to 320 degree F and grease an Air fryer basket.
2. Spray the tomato halves evenly with olive oil cooking spray and season with salt, black pepper and basil.
3. Arrange the tomato halves into the Air fryer basket, cut sides up.
4. Cook for about 10 minutes and dish out onto serving plates.

Nutrition Info: Calories: 22, Fat: 4.8g, Carbohydrates: 4.8g, Sugar: 3.2g, Protein: 1.1g, Sodium: 84mg

134.Salsa Stuffed Eggplants

Servings: 2
Cooking Time: 25 Minutes
Ingredients:

- 1 large eggplant
- 8 cherry tomatoes, quartered
- ½ tablespoon fresh parsley
- 2 teaspoons olive oil, divided
- 2 teaspoons fresh lemon juice, divided
- 2 tablespoons tomato salsa
- Salt and black pepper, as required

Directions:

1. Preheat the Air fryer to 390 degree F and grease an Air fryer basket.
2. Arrange the eggplant into the Air fryer basket and cook for about 15 minutes.
3. Cut the eggplant in half lengthwise and drizzle evenly with one teaspoon of oil.
4. Set the Air fryer to 355 degree F and arrange the eggplant into the Air fryer basket, cut-side up.
5. Cook for another 10 minutes and dish out in a bowl.

6. Scoop out the flesh from the eggplant and transfer into a bowl.
7. Stir in the tomatoes, salsa, parsley, salt, black pepper, remaining oil, and lemon juice.
8. Squeeze lemon juice on the eggplant halves and stuff with the salsa mixture to serve.
Nutrition Info: Calories: 192, Fat: 6.1g, Carbohydrates: 33.8g, Sugar: 20.4g, Protein: 6.9g, Sodium: 204mg

135.Lamb Skewers

Servings: 4
Cooking Time: 20 Minutes
Ingredients:
- 2 lb. lamb meat; cubed
- 2 red bell peppers; cut into medium pieces
- ¼ cup olive oil
- 2 tbsp. lemon juice
- 1 tbsp. oregano; dried
- 1 tbsp. red vinegar
- 1 tbsp. garlic; minced
- ½ tsp. rosemary; dried
- A pinch of salt and black pepper

Directions:
1. Take a bowl and mix all the ingredients and toss them well.
2. Thread the lamb and bell peppers on skewers, place them in your air fryer's basket and cook at 380°F for 10 minutes on each side. Divide between plates and serve with a side salad
Nutrition Info: Calories: 274; Fat: 12g; Fiber: 3g; Carbs: 6g; Protein: 16g

136.Cheese Zucchini Boats

Servings: 2
Cooking Time: 20 Minutes
Ingredients:
- 2 medium zucchinis
- ¼ cup full-fat ricotta cheese
- ¼ cup shredded mozzarella cheese
- ¼ cup low-carb, no-sugar-added pasta sauce.
- 2 tbsp. grated vegetarian Parmesan cheese
- 1 tbsp. avocado oil
- ¼ tsp. garlic powder.
- ½ tsp. dried parsley.
- ¼ tsp. dried oregano.

Directions:
1. Cut off 1-inch from the top and bottom of each zucchini.
2. Slice zucchini in half lengthwise and use a spoon to scoop out a bit of the inside, making room for filling. Brush with oil and spoon 2 tbsp. pasta sauce into each shell

3. Take a medium bowl, mix ricotta, mozzarella, oregano, garlic powder and parsley
4. Spoon the mixture into each zucchini shell. Place stuffed zucchini shells into the air fryer basket.
5. Adjust the temperature to 350 Degrees F and set the timer for 20 minutes
6. To remove from the fryer basket, use tongs or a spatula and carefully lift out. Top with Parmesan. Serve immediately.
Nutrition Info: Calories: 215; Protein: 15g; Fiber: 7g; Fat: 19g; Carbs: 3g

137.Roasted Lamb

Servings: 4
Cooking Time: 1 Hour 30 Minutes
Ingredients:
- 2½ pounds half lamb leg roast, slits carved
- 2 garlic cloves, sliced into smaller slithers
- 1 tablespoon dried rosemary
- 1 tablespoon olive oil
- Cracked Himalayan rock salt and cracked peppercorns, to taste

Directions:
1. Preheat the Air fryer to 400 degree F and grease an Air fryer basket.
2. Insert the garlic slithers in the slits and brush with rosemary, oil, salt, and black pepper.
3. Arrange the lamb in the Air fryer basket and cook for about 15 minutes.
4. Set the Air fryer to 350 degree F on the Roast mode and cook for 1 hour and 15 minutes.
5. Dish out the lamb chops and serve hot.
Nutrition Info: Calories: 246, Fat: 7.4g, Carbohydrates: 9.4g, Sugar: 6.5g, Protein: 37.2g, Sodium: 353mg

138.Spicy Paprika Steak

Servings: 2
Cooking Time: 20 Minutes
Ingredients:
- 1/2 Ancho chili pepper, soaked in hot water before using
- 1 tablespoon brandy
- 2 teaspoons smoked paprika
- 1 1/2 tablespoons olive oil
- 2 beef steaks
- Kosher salt, to taste
- 1 teaspoon ground allspice
- 3 cloves garlic, sliced

Directions:
1. Sprinkle the beef steaks with salt, paprika, and allspice. Add the steak to a baking dish that fits your fryer. Scatter the sliced garlic over the top.

2. Now, drizzle it with brandy and olive oil; spread minced Ancho chili pepper over the top.
3. Bake at 385 degrees F for 14 minutes, turning halfway through. Serve warm.
Nutrition Info: 450 Calories; 26g Fat; 4g Carbs; 58g Protein; 3g Sugars; 3g Fiber

139.Lemon Garlic Shrimps

Servings: 2
Cooking Time: 8 Minutes
Ingredients:
- ¾ pound medium shrimp, peeled and deveined
- 1½ tablespoons fresh lemon juice
- 1 tablespoon olive oil
- 1 teaspoon lemon pepper
- ¼ teaspoon paprika
- ¼ teaspoon garlic powder

Directions:
1. Preheat the Air fryer to 400 degree F and grease an Air fryer basket.
2. Mix lemon juice, olive oil, lemon pepper, paprika and garlic powder in a large bowl.
3. Stir in the shrimp and toss until well combined.
4. Arrange shrimp into the Air fryer basket in a single layer and cook for about 8 minutes.
5. Dish out the shrimp in serving plates and serve warm.
Nutrition Info: Calories: 260, Fat: 12.4g, Carbohydrates: 0.3g, Sugar: 0.1g, Protein: 35.6g, Sodium: 619mg

140.Spiced Salmon Kebabs

Servings: 3
Cooking Time: 15 Minutes
Ingredients:
- 2 tablespoons chopped fresh oregano
- 2 teaspoons sesame seeds
- 1 teaspoon ground cumin
- Salt and pepper to taste
- 1 ½ pounds salmon fillets
- 2 tablespoons olive oil
- 2 lemons, sliced into rounds

Directions:
1. Place the instant pot air fryer lid on and preheat the instant pot at 390 degrees F.
2. Place the grill pan accessory in the instant pot.
3. Create dry rub by combining the oregano, sesame seeds, cumin, salt, and pepper.
4. Rub the salmon fillets with the dry rub and brush with oil.
5. Place on the grill pan, close the air fryer lid and grill the salmon for 15 minutes.
6. Serve with lemon slices once cooked.

Nutrition Info: Calories per serving 447 ; Carbs: 4.1g; Protein:47.6 g; Fat:26.6 g

141.Carrot Beef Cake

Servings: 10
Cooking Time: 60 Minutes
Ingredients:
- 3 eggs, beaten
- 1/2 cup almond milk
- 1-oz. onion soup mix
- 1 cup dry bread crumbs
- 2 cups shredded carrots
- 2 lbs. lean ground beef
- 1/2-lb. ground pork

Directions:
1. Thoroughly mix ground beef with carrots and all other ingredients in a bowl.
2. Grease a meatloaf pan with oil or butter and spread the minced beef in the pan.
3. Press "Power Button" of Air Fry Oven and turn the dial to select the "Bake" mode.
4. Press the Time button and again turn the dial to set the cooking time to 60 minutes.
5. Now push the Temp button and rotate the dial to set the temperature at 350 degrees F.
6. Once preheated, place the beef baking pan in the oven and close its lid.
7. Slice and serve.
Nutrition Info: Calories: 212 Cal Total Fat: 11.8 g Saturated Fat: 2.2 g Cholesterol: 23 mg Sodium: 321 mg Total Carbs: 14.6 g Fiber: 4.4 g Sugar: 8 g Protein: 17.3 g

142.Air Fryer Buffalo Mushroom Poppers

Servings: 8
Cooking Time: 50 Minutes
Ingredients:
- 1 pound fresh whole button mushrooms
- 1/2 teaspoon kosher salt
- 3 tablespoons 1/3-less-fat cream cheese,
- 1/4 cup all-purpose flour
- Softened 1 jalapeño chile, seeded and minced
- Cooking spray
- 1/4 teaspoon black pepper
- 1 cup panko breadcrumbs
- 2 large eggs, lightly beaten
- 1/4 cup buffalo-style hot sauce
- 2 tablespoons chopped fresh chives
- 1/2 cup low-fat buttermilk
- 1/2 cup plain fat-free yogurt
- 2 ounces blue cheese, crumbled (about 1/2 cup)
- 3 tablespoons apple cider vinegar

Directions:

1. Remove stems from mushroom caps, chop stems and set caps aside. Stir together chopped mushroom stems, cream cheese, jalapeño, salt, and pepper. Stuff about 1 teaspoon of the mixture into each mushroom cap, rounding the filling to form a smooth ball.
2. Place panko in a bowl, place flour in a second bowl, and eggs in a third Coat mushrooms in flour, dip in egg mixture, and dredge in panko, pressing to adhere. Spray mushrooms well with cooking spray.
3. Place half of the mushrooms in air fryer basket, and cook for 20 minutes at 350°F. Transfer cooked mushrooms to a large bowl. Drizzle buffalo sauce over mushrooms; toss to coat then sprinkle with chives.
4. Stir buttermilk, yogurt, blue cheese, and cider vinegar in a small bowl. Serve mushroom poppers with blue cheese sauce.

Nutrition Info: Calories 133 Fat 4g Saturated fat 2g Unsaturated fat 2g Protein 7g Carbohydrate 16g Fiber 1g Sugars 3g Sodium 485mg Calcium 10% DV Potassium 7% DV

143.Keto Lamb Kleftiko

Servings: 6
Cooking Time: 30 Minutes
Ingredients:
- 2 oz. garlic clove, peeled
- 1 tablespoon dried oregano
- ½ lemon
- ¼ tablespoon ground cinnamon
- 3 tablespoon butter, frozen
- 18 oz. leg of lamb
- 1 cup heavy cream
- 1 teaspoon bay leaf
- 1 teaspoon dried mint
- 1 tablespoon olive oil

Directions:
1. Crush the garlic cloves and combine them with the dried oregano, and ground cinnamon. Mix it.
2. Then chop the lemon.
3. Sprinkle the leg of lamb with the crushed garlic mixture.
4. Then rub it with the chopped lemon.
5. Combine the heavy cream, bay leaf, and dried mint together.
6. Whisk the mixture well.
7. After this, add the olive oil and whisk it one more time more.
8. Then pour the cream mixture on the leg of lamb and stir it carefully.
9. Leave the leg of lamb for 10 minutes to marinate.
10. Preheat the air fryer to 380 F.
11. Chop the butter and sprinkle the marinated lamb.

12. Then place the leg of lamb in the air fryer basket tray and sprinkle it with the remaining cream mixture.
13. Then sprinkle the meat with the chopped butter.
14. Cook the meat for 30 minutes.
15. When the time is over – remove the meat from the air fryer and sprinkle it gently with the remaining cream mixture.
16. Serve it!

Nutrition Info: calories 318, fat 21.9, fiber 0.9, carbs 4.9, protein 25.1

144.Oven-fried Herbed Chicken

Servings: 2
Cooking Time: 15 Minutes
Ingredients:
- 1/2 cup buttermilk
- 2 cloves garlic, minced
- 1-1/2 teaspoons salt
- 1 tablespoon oil
- 1/2 pound boneless, skinless chicken breasts
- 1 cup rolled oats
- 1/2 teaspoon red pepper flakes
- 1/2 cup grated parmesan cheese
- 1/4 cup fresh basil leaves or rosemary needles
- Olive oil spray

Directions:
1. Mix together buttermilk, oil, 1/2 teaspoon salt, and garlic in a shallow bowl.
2. Roll chicken in buttermilk and refrigerate in bowl overnight.
3. Preheat your toaster oven to 425°F.
4. Mix together the oats, red pepper, salt, parmesan, and basil, and mix roughly to break up oats.
5. Place the mixture on a plate.
6. Remove the chicken from the buttermilk mixture and let any excess drip off.
7. Roll the chicken in the oat mixture and transfer to a baking sheet lightly coated with olive oil spray.
8. Spray the chicken with oil spray and bake for 15 minutes.

Nutrition Info: Calories: 651, Sodium: 713 mg, Dietary Fiber: 4.4 g, Total Fat: 31.2 g, Total Carbs: 34.1 g, Protein: 59.5 g.

145.Crispy Scallops

Servings: 4
Cooking Time: 6 Minutes
Ingredients:
- 18 sea scallops, cleaned and patted very dry
- 1/8 cup all-purpose flour
- 1 tablespoon 2% milk

45

- ½ egg
- ¼ cup cornflakes, crushed
- ½ teaspoon paprika
- Salt and black pepper, as required

Directions:
1. Preheat the Air fryer to 400 degree F and grease an Air fryer basket.
2. Mix flour, paprika, salt, and black pepper in a bowl.
3. Whisk egg with milk in another bowl and place the cornflakes in a third bowl.
4. Coat each scallop with the flour mixture, dip into the egg mixture and finally, dredge in the cornflakes.
5. Arrange scallops in the Air fryer basket and cook for about 6 minutes.
6. Dish out the scallops in a platter and serve hot.

Nutrition Info: Calories: 150, Fat: 1.7g, Carbohydrates: 8g, Sugar: 0.4g, Protein: 24g, Sodium: 278mg

146.Chat Masala Grilled Snapper

Servings: 5
Cooking Time: 25 Minutes
Ingredients:
- 2 ½ pounds whole fish
- Salt to taste
- 1/3 cup chat masala
- 3 tablespoons fresh lime juice
- 5 tablespoons olive oil

Directions:
1. Place the instant pot air fryer lid on and preheat the instant pot at 390 degrees F.
2. Place the grill pan accessory in the instant pot.
3. Season the fish with salt, chat masala and lime juice.
4. Brush with oil
5. Place the fish on a foil basket and place it inside the grill.
6. Close the air fryer lid and cook for 25 minutes.

Nutrition Info: Calories:308; Carbs: 0.7g; Protein: 35.2g; Fat: 17.4g

147.Pork Chops With Chicory Treviso

Servings: 2
Cooking Time: 0-15;
Ingredients:
- 4 pork chops
- 40g butter
- Flour to taste
- 1 chicory stalk
- Salt to taste

Directions:

1. Cut the chicory into small pieces. Place the butter and chicory in pieces on the basket of the air fryer previously preheated at 1800C and brown for 2 min.
2. Add the previously floured and salted pork slices (directly over the chicory), simmer for 6 minutes turning them over after 3 minutes.
3. Remove the slices and place them on a serving plate, covering them with the rest of the red chicory juice collected at the bottom of the basket.

Nutrition Info: Calories 504, Fat 33, Carbohydrates 0g, Sugars 0g, Protein 42g, Cholesterol 130mg

148.Baked Veggie Egg Rolls

Servings: 2
Cooking Time: 20 Minutes
Ingredients:
- 1/2 tablespoon olive or vegetable oil
- 2 cups thinly-sliced chard
- 1/4 cup grated carrot
- 1/2 cup chopped pea pods
- 3 shiitake mushrooms
- 2 scallions
- 2 medium cloves garlic
- 1/2 tablespoon fresh ginger
- 1/2 tablespoon soy sauce
- 6 egg roll wrappers
- Olive oil spray for cookie sheet and egg rolls

Directions:
1. Start by mincing mushrooms, garlic, and ginger and slicing scallions.
2. Heat oil on medium heat in a medium skillet and char peas, carrots, scallions, and mushrooms.
3. Cook 3 minutes, then add ginger. Stir in soy sauce and remove from heat.
4. Preheat toaster oven to 400°F and spray cookie sheet. Spoon even portions of vegetable mix over each egg roll wrapper, and wrap them up.
5. Place egg rolls on cookie sheet and spray with olive oil. Bake for 20 minutes until egg roll shells are browned.

Nutrition Info: Calories: 421, Sodium: 1166 mg, Dietary Fiber: 8.2 g, Total Fat: 7.7 g, Total Carbs: 76.9 g, Protein: 13.7 g.

149.One-pan Shrimp And Chorizo Mix Grill

Servings: 4
Cooking Time: 15 Minutes
Ingredients:
- 1 ½ pounds large shrimps, peeled and deveined
- Salt and pepper to taste
- 6 links fresh chorizo sausage
- 2 bunches asparagus spears, trimmed

- Lime wedges

Directions:
1. Place the instant pot air fryer lid on and preheat the instant pot at 390 degrees F.
2. Place the grill pan accessory in the instant pot.
3. Season the shrimps with salt and pepper to taste. Set aside.
4. Place the chorizo on the grill pan and the sausage.
5. Place the asparagus on top.
6. Close the air fryer lid and grill for 15 minutes.
7. Serve with lime wedges.

Nutrition Info: Calories:124 ; Carbs: 9.4g; Protein: 8.2g; Fat: 7.1g

150.Air Fryer Roasted Broccoli

Servings: 4
Cooking Time: 10 Minutes
Ingredients:
- 1 tsp. herbes de provence seasoning (optional)
- 4 cups fresh broccoli
- 1 tablespoon olive oil
- Salt and pepper to taste

Directions:
1. Drizzle or spray broccoli with olive and sprinkle seasoning throughout
2. Spray air fryer basket with cooking oil, place broccoli and cook for 5-8 minutes on 360F
3. Open air fryer and examine broccoli after 5 minutes because different fryer brands cook at different rates.

Nutrition Info: Calories 61 Fat 4g protein 3g net carbs 4g

151.Crumbly Oat Meatloaf

Servings: 8
Cooking Time: 60 Minutes
Ingredients:
- 2 lbs. ground beef
- 1 cup of salsa
- 3/4 cup Quaker Oats
- 1/2 cup chopped onion
- 1 large egg, beaten
- 1 tablespoon Worcestershire sauce
- Salt and black pepper to taste

Directions:
1. Thoroughly mix ground beef with salsa, oats, onion, egg, and all the ingredients in a bowl.
2. Grease a meatloaf pan with oil or butter and spread the minced beef in the pan.
3. Press "Power Button" of Air Fry Oven and turn the dial to select the "Bake" mode.

4. Press the Time button and again turn the dial to set the cooking time to 60 minutes.
5. Now push the Temp button and rotate the dial to set the temperature at 350 degrees F.
6. Once preheated, place the beef baking pan in the oven and close its lid.
7. Slice and serve.

Nutrition Info: Calories: 412 Cal Total Fat: 24.8 g Saturated Fat: 12.4 g Cholesterol: 3 mg Sodium: 132 mg Total Carbs: 43.8 g Fiber: 3.9 g Sugar: 2.5 g Protein: 18.9 g

152.Roasted Garlic Zucchini Rolls

Servings: 4
Cooking Time: 20 Minutes
Ingredients:
- 2 medium zucchinis
- ½ cup full-fat ricotta cheese
- ¼ white onion; peeled. And diced
- 2 cups spinach; chopped
- ¼ cup heavy cream
- ½ cup sliced baby portobello mushrooms
- ¾ cup shredded mozzarella cheese, divided.
- 2 tbsp. unsalted butter.
- 2 tbsp. vegetable broth.
- ½ tsp. finely minced roasted garlic
- ¼ tsp. dried oregano.
- ⅛ tsp. xanthan gum
- ¼ tsp. salt
- ½ tsp. garlic powder.

Directions:
1. Using a mandoline or sharp knife, slice zucchini into long strips lengthwise. Place strips between paper towels to absorb moisture. Set aside
2. In a medium saucepan over medium heat, melt butter. Add onion and sauté until fragrant. Add garlic and sauté 30 seconds.
3. Pour in heavy cream, broth and xanthan gum. Turn off heat and whisk mixture until it begins to thicken, about 3 minutes.
4. Take a medium bowl, add ricotta, salt, garlic powder and oregano and mix well. Fold in spinach, mushrooms and ½ cup mozzarella
5. Pour half of the sauce into a 6-inch round baking pan. To assemble the rolls, place two strips of zucchini on a work surface. Spoon 2 tbsp. of ricotta mixture onto the slices and roll up. Place seam side down on top of sauce. Repeat with remaining ingredients
6. Pour remaining sauce over the rolls and sprinkle with remaining mozzarella. Cover with foil and place into the air fryer basket. Adjust the temperature to 350 Degrees F and set the timer for 20 minutes. In the last 5 minutes, remove the foil to brown the cheese. Serve immediately.

Nutrition Info: Calories: 245; Protein: 15g; Fiber: 8g; Fat: 19g; Carbs: 1g

Nutrition Info: 292 Calories; 11g Fat; 1g Carbs; 22g Protein; 9g Sugars; 6g Fiber

153.Buttered Scallops

Servings: 2
Cooking Time: 4 Minutes
Ingredients:
- ¾ pound sea scallops, cleaned and patted very dry
- 1 tablespoon butter, melted
- ½ tablespoon fresh thyme, minced
- Salt and black pepper, as required

Directions:
1. Preheat the Air fryer to 390 degree F and grease an Air fryer basket.
2. Mix scallops, butter, thyme, salt, and black pepper in a bowl.
3. Arrange scallops in the Air fryer basket and cook for about 4 minutes.
4. Dish out the scallops in a platter and serve hot.
Nutrition Info: Calories: 202, Fat: 7.1g, Carbohydrates: 4.4g, Sugar: 0g, Protein: 28.7g, Sodium: 393mg

154.Greek-style Monkfish With Vegetables

Servings: 2
Cooking Time: 20 Minutes
Ingredients:
- 2 teaspoons olive oil
- 1 cup celery, sliced
- 2 bell peppers, sliced
- 1 teaspoon dried thyme
- 1/2 teaspoon dried marjoram
- 1/2 teaspoon dried rosemary
- 2 monkfish fillets
- 1 tablespoon soy sauce
- 2 tablespoons lime juice
- Coarse salt and ground black pepper, to taste
- 1 teaspoon cayenne pepper
- 1/2 cup Kalamata olives, pitted and sliced

Directions:
1. In a nonstick skillet, heat the olive oil for 1 minute. Once hot, sauté the celery and peppers until tender, about 4 minutes. Sprinkle with thyme, marjoram, and rosemary and set aside.
2. Toss the fish fillets with the soy sauce, lime juice, salt, black pepper, and cayenne pepper. Place the fish fillets in a lightly greased cooking basket and bake at 390 degrees F for 8 minutes.
3. Turn them over, add the olives, and cook an additional 4 minutes. Serve with the sautéed vegetables on the side.

155.Flank Steak Beef

Servings: 4
Cooking Time: 20 Minutes
Ingredients:
- 1 pound flank steaks, sliced
- ¼ cup xanthum gum
- 2 teaspoon vegetable oil
- ½ teaspoon ginger
- ½ cup soy sauce
- 1 tablespoon garlic, minced
- ½ cup water
- ¾ cup swerve, packed

Directions:
1. Preheat the Air fryer to 390 degree F and grease an Air fryer basket.
2. Coat the steaks with xanthum gum on both the sides and transfer into the Air fryer basket.
3. Cook for about 10 minutes and dish out in a platter.
4. Meanwhile, cook rest of the ingredients for the sauce in a saucepan.
5. Bring to a boil and pour over the steak slices to serve.
Nutrition Info: Calories: 372, Fat: 11.8g, Carbohydrates: 1.8g, Sugar: 27.3g, Protein: 34g, Sodium: 871mg

156.Chicken Lasagna With Eggplants

Servings: 10
Cooking Time: 17 Minutes
Ingredients:
- 6 oz Cheddar cheese, shredded
- 7 oz Parmesan cheese, shredded
- 2 eggplants
- 1-pound ground chicken
- 1 teaspoon paprika
- 1 teaspoon salt
- ½ teaspoon cayenne pepper
- ½ cup heavy cream
- 2 teaspoon butter
- 4 oz chive stems, diced

Directions:
1. Take the air fryer basket tray and spread it with the butter.
2. Then peel the eggplants and slice them.
3. Separate the sliced eggplants into 3 parts.
4. Combine the ground chicken with the paprika, salt, cayenne pepper, and diced chives.
5. Mix the mixture up.

6. Separate the ground chicken mixture into 2 parts.
7. Make the layer of the first part of the sliced eggplant in the air fryer basket tray.
8. Then make the layer of the ground chicken mixture.
9. After this, sprinkle the ground chicken layer with the half of the shredded Cheddar cheese,
10. Then cover the cheese with the second part of the sliced eggplant.
11. The next step is to make the layer of the ground chicken and all shredded Cheddar cheese,
12. Cover the cheese layer with the last part of the sliced eggplants.
13. Then sprinkle the eggplants with shredded Parmesan cheese.
14. Pour the heavy cream and add butter.
15. Preheat the air fryer to 365 F.
16. Cook the lasagna for 17 minutes.
17. When the time is over – let the lasagna chill gently.
18. Serve it!
Nutrition Info: calories 291, fat 17.6, fiber 4.6, carbs 7.8, protein 27.4

157.Cheese And Garlic Stuffed Chicken Breasts

Servings: 2
Cooking Time: 20 Minutes
Ingredients:
- 1/2 cup Cottage cheese 2 eggs, beaten
- 2 medium-sized chicken breasts, halved
- 2 tablespoons fresh coriander, chopped 1tsp. fine sea salt
- Seasoned breadcrumbs
- 1/3 tsp. freshly ground black pepper, to savor 3 cloves garlic, finely minced

Directions:
1. Firstly, flatten out the chicken breast using a meat tenderizer.
2. In a medium-sized mixing dish, combine the Cottage cheese with the garlic, coriander, salt, and black pepper.
3. Spread 1/3 of the mixture over the first chicken breast. Repeat with the remaining ingredients. Roll the chicken around the filling; make sure to secure with toothpicks.
4. Now, whisk the egg in a shallow bowl. In another shallow bowl, combine the salt, ground black pepper, and seasoned breadcrumbs.
5. Coat the chicken breasts with the whisked egg; now, roll them in the breadcrumbs.
6. Cook in the air fryer cooking basket at 365 °F for 22 minutes. Serve immediately.

Nutrition Info: 424 Calories; 24.5g Fat; 7.5g Carbs; 43.4g Protein; 5.3g Sugars

158.Korean Beef Bowl

Servings: 4
Cooking Time: 18 Minutes
Ingredients:
- 1 tablespoon minced garlic
- 1 teaspoon ground ginger
- 4 oz chive stems, chopped
- 2 tablespoon apple cider vinegar
- 1 teaspoon stevia extract
- 1 tablespoon flax seeds
- 1 teaspoon olive oil
- 1 teaspoon olive oil
- 1-pound ground beef
- 4 tablespoon chicken stock

Directions:
1. Sprinkle the ground beef with the apple cider vinegar and stir the meat with the help of the spoon.
2. After this, sprinkle the ground beef with the ground ginger, minced garlic, and olive oil.
3. Mix it up.
4. Preheat the air fryer to 370 F.
5. Put the ground beef in the air fryer basket tray and cook it for 8 minutes.
6. After this, stir the ground beef carefully and sprinkle with the chopped chives, flax seeds, olive oil, and chicken stock.
7. Mix the dish up and cook it for 10 minutes more.
8. When the time is over – stir the dish carefully.
9. Serve Korean beef bowl immediately.
10. Enjoy!
Nutrition Info: calories 258, fat 10.1, fiber 1.2, carbs 4.2, protein 35.3

159.Sautéed Green Beans

Servings: 2
Cooking Time: 10 Minutes
Ingredients:
- 8 ounces fresh green beans, trimmed and cut in half
- 1 teaspoon sesame oil
- 1 tablespoon soy sauce

Directions:
1. Preheat the Air fryer to 390F and grease an Air fryer basket.
2. Mix green beans, soy sauce, and sesame oil in a bowl and toss to coat well.
3. Arrange green beans into the Air fryer basket and cook for about 10 minutes, tossing once in between.
4. Dish out onto serving plates and serve hot.

Nutrition Info: Calories: 59, Fats: 2.4g, Carbohydrates: 59g, Sugar: 1.7g, Proteins: 2.6g, Sodium: 458mg

160.Spicy Cauliflower Rice

Servings: 2
Cooking Time: 22 Minutes
Ingredients:
- 1 cauliflower head, cut into florets 1/2 tsp cumin
- 1/2 tsp chili powder
- 6 onion spring, chopped 2 jalapenos, chopped
- 4 tbsp olive oil
- 1 zucchini, trimmed and cut into cubes 1/2 tsp paprika
- 1/2 tsp garlic powder 1/2 tsp cayenne pepper 1/2 tsp pepper
- 1/2 tsp salt

Directions:
1. Preheat the air fryer to 370 F.
2. Add cauliflower florets into the food processor and process until it looks like rice.
3. Transfer cauliflower rice into the air fryer baking pan and drizzle with half oil.
4. Place pan in the air fryer and cook for 12 minutes, stir halfway through.
5. Heat remaining oil in a small pan over medium heat.
6. Add zucchini and cook for 5-8 minutes.
7. Add onion and jalapenos and cook for 5 minutes.
8. Add spices and stir well. Set aside.
9. Add cauliflower rice in the zucchini mixture and stir well.
10. Serve and enjoy.
Nutrition Info: Calories 254 Fat 28 g Carbohydrates 12.3 g Sugar 5 g

161.Broccoli Stuffed Peppers

Servings: 2
Cooking Time: 40 Minutes
Ingredients:
- 4 eggs
- 1/2 cup cheddar cheese, grated
- 2 bell peppers, cut in half and remove seeds 1/2 tsp garlic powder
- 1 tsp dried thyme
- 1/4 cup feta cheese, crumbled 1/2 cup broccoli, cooked
- 1/4 tsp pepper 1/2 tsp salt

Directions:
1. Preheat the air fryer to 325 F.
2. Stuff feta and broccoli into the bell peppers halved.

3. Beat egg in a bowl with seasoning and pour egg mixture into the pepper halved over feta and broccoli.
4. Place bell pepper halved into the air fryer basket and cook for 35-40 minutes.
5. Top with grated cheddar cheese and cook until cheese melted.
6. Serve and enjoy.
Nutrition Info: Calories 340 Fat 22 g Carbohydrates 12 g Sugar 8.2 g Protein 22 g Cholesterol 374 mg

162.Effortless Beef Schnitzel

Servings: 2
Cooking Time: 25 Minutes
Ingredients:
- 2 tbsp vegetable oil
- 2 oz breadcrumbs
- 1 whole egg, whisked
- 1 thin beef schnitzel, cut into strips
- 1 whole lemon

Directions:
1. Preheat your fryer to 356 F. In a bowl, add breadcrumbs and oil and stir well to get a loose mixture. Dip schnitzel in egg, then dip in breadcrumbs coat well. Place the prepared schnitzel your Air Fryer's cooking basket and cook for 12 minutes. Serve with a drizzle of lemon juice.
Nutrition Info: 346 Calories; 11g Fat; 4g Carbs; 32g Protein; 1g Sugars; 1g Fiber

163.Ham Rolls

Servings: 4
Cooking Time: 15 Minutes
Ingredients:
- 12-ounce refrigerated pizza crust, rolled into ¼ inch thickness
- 1/3 pound cooked ham, sliced
- ¾ cup Mozzarella cheese, shredded
- 3 cups Colby cheese, shredded
- 3-ounce roasted red bell peppers
- 1 tablespoon olive oil

Directions:
1. Preheat the Air fryer to 360 degree F and grease an Air fryer basket.
2. Arrange the ham, cheeses and roasted peppers over one side of dough and fold to seal.
3. Brush the dough evenly with olive oil and cook for about 15 minutes, flipping twice in between.
4. Dish out in a platter and serve warm.
Nutrition Info: Calories: 594, Fat: 35.8g, Carbohydrates: 35.4g, Sugar: 2.8g, Protein: 33g, Sodium: 1545mg

164. Salmon Steak Grilled With Cilantro Garlic Sauce

Servings: 2
Cooking Time: 15 Minutes
Ingredients:

- 2 salmon steaks
- Salt and pepper to taste
- 2 tablespoons vegetable oil
- 2 cloves of garlic, minced
- 1 cup cilantro leaves
- ½ cup Greek yogurt
- 1 teaspoon honey

Directions:
1. Place the instant pot air fryer lid on and preheat the instant pot at 390 degrees F.
2. Place the grill pan accessory in the instant pot.
3. Season the salmon steaks with salt and pepper. Brush with oil.
4. Place on the grill pan, close the air fryer lid and grill for 15 minutes and make sure to flip halfway through the cooking time.
5. In a food processor, mix the garlic, cilantro leaves, yogurt, and honey. Season with salt and pepper to taste. Pulse until smooth.
6. Serve the salmon steaks with the cilantro sauce.
Nutrition Info: Calories: 485; Carbs: 6.3g; Protein: 47.6g; Fat: 29.9g

165. Healthy Mama Meatloaf

Servings: 8
Cooking Time: 40 Minutes
Ingredients:

- 1 tablespoon olive oil
- 1 green bell pepper, diced
- 1/2 cup diced sweet onion
- 1/2 teaspoon minced garlic
- 1-lb. ground beef
- 1 cup whole wheat bread crumbs
- 2 large eggs
- 3/4 cup shredded carrot
- 3/4 cup shredded zucchini
- salt and ground black pepper to taste
- 1/4 cup ketchup, or to taste

Directions:
1. Thoroughly mix ground beef with egg, onion, garlic, crumbs, and all the ingredients in a bowl.
2. Grease a meatloaf pan with oil or butter and spread the minced beef in the pan.
3. Press "Power Button" of Air Fry Oven and turn the dial to select the "Bake" mode.
4. Press the Time button and again turn the dial to set the cooking time to 40 minutes.
5. Now push the Temp button and rotate the dial to set the temperature at 375 degrees F.

6. Once preheated, place the beef baking pan in the oven and close its lid.
7. Slice and serve.
Nutrition Info: Calories: 322 Cal Total Fat: 11.8 g Saturated Fat: 2.2 g Cholesterol: 56 mg Sodium: 321 mg Total Carbs: 14.6 g Fiber: 4.4 g Sugar: 8 g Protein: 17.3 g

166. Chili Pepper Lamb Chops

Servings: 6
Cooking Time: 10 Minutes
Ingredients:

- 21 oz. lamb chops
- 1 teaspoon chili pepper
- ½ teaspoon chili flakes
- 1 teaspoon onion powder
- 1 teaspoon garlic powder
- 1 teaspoon cayenne pepper
- 1 tablespoon olive oil
- 1 tablespoon butter
- ½ teaspoon lime zest

Directions:
1. Melt the butter and combine it with the olive oil.
2. Whisk the liquid and add chili pepper, chili flakes, onion powder, garlic powder, cayenne pepper, and lime zest.
3. Whisk it well
4. Then sprinkle the lamb chops with the prepared oily marinade.
5. Leave the meat for at least 5 minutes in the fridge.
6. Preheat the air fryer to 400 F.
7. Place the marinated lamb chops in the air fryer and cook them for 5 minutes.
8. After this, open the air fryer and turn the lamb chops into another side.
9. Cook the lamb chops for 5 minutes more.
10. When the meat is cooked – transfer it to the serving plates.
11. Enjoy!
Nutrition Info: calories 227, fat 11.6, fiber 0.2, carbs 1, protein 28.1

167. Lemony Green Beans

Servings: 3
Cooking Time: 12 Minutes
Ingredients:

- 1 pound green beans, trimmed and halved
- 1 teaspoon butter, melted
- 1 tablespoon fresh lemon juice
- ¼ teaspoon garlic powder

Directions:

1. Preheat the Air fryer to 400F and grease an Air fryer basket.
2. Mix all the ingredients in a bowl and toss to coat well.
3. Arrange the green beans into the Air fryer basket and cook for about 12 minutes.
4. Dish out in a serving plate and serve hot.
Nutrition Info: Calories: 60, Fat: 1.5g, Carbohydrates: 11.1g, Sugar: 2.3g, Protein: 2.8g, Sodium: 70mg

168.Asparagus Frittata

Servings: 4
Cooking Time: 10 Minutes
Ingredients:
- 6 eggs
- 3 mushrooms, sliced
- 10 asparagus, chopped 1/4 cup half and half
- 2 tsp butter, melted
- 1 cup mozzarella cheese, shredded 1 tsp pepper
- 1 tsp salt

Directions:
1. Toss mushrooms and asparagus with melted butter and add into the air fryer basket.
2. Cook mushrooms and asparagus at 350 F for 5 minutes. Shake basket twice.
3. Meanwhile, in a bowl, whisk together eggs, half and half, pepper, and salt.
4. Transfer cook mushrooms and asparagus into the air fryer baking dish.
5. Pour egg mixture over mushrooms and asparagus.
6. Place dish in the air fryer and cook at 350 F for 5 minutes or until eggs are set.
7. Slice and serve.
Nutrition Info: Calories 211 Fat 13 g Carbohydrates 4 g Sugar 1 g Protein 16 g Cholesterol 272 mg

169.Cheddar & Dijon Tuna Melt

Servings: 1
Cooking Time: 7 Minutes
Ingredients:
- 1 (6-ounce) can tuna, drained and flaked
- 2 tablespoons mayonnaise
- 1 pinch salt
- 1 teaspoon balsamic vinegar
- 1 teaspoon Dijon mustard
- 2 slices whole wheat bread
- 2 teaspoons chopped dill pickle
- 1/4 cup shredded sharp cheddar cheese

Directions:
1. Start by preheating toaster oven to 375°F.
2. Put bread in toaster while it warms.

3. Mix together tuna, mayo, salt, vinegar, mustard, and pickle in a small bowl.
4. Remove bread from oven and put tuna mixture on one side and the cheese on the other.
5. Return to toaster oven and bake for 7 minutes.
6. Combine slices, then cut and serve.
Nutrition Info: Calories: 688, Sodium: 1024 mg, Dietary Fiber: 4.1 g, Total Fat: 35.0 g, Total Carbs: 31.0 g, Protein: 59.9 g.

170.Rigatoni With Roasted Broccoli And Chick Peas

Servings: 4
Cooking Time: 10 Minutes
Ingredients:
- 1 can anchovies packed in oil
- 4 cloves garlic, chopped
- 1 can chickpeas
- 1 chicken bouillon cube
- 1 pound broccoli, cut into small florets
- 1/2 pound whole wheat rigatoni
- 1/2 cup grated Romano cheese

Directions:
1. Drain and chop anchovies (set aside oil for later use), and cut broccoli into small florets.
2. Preheat toaster oven to 450°F.
3. In a shallow sauce pan, sauté anchovies in their oil, with garlic, until the garlic browns.
4. Drain the chickpeas, saving the canned liquid.
5. Add the chickpea liquid and bouillon to the anchovies, stir until bouillon dissolves.
6. Pour anchovy mix into a roasting pan and add broccoli and chickpeas.
7. Roast for 20 minutes.
8. While the veggies roast, cook rigatoni per package directions; drain the pasta, saving one cup of water.
9. Add the pasta to the anchovy mix and roast for another 10 minutes. Add reserved water, stirring in a little at a time until the pasta reaches the desired consistency.
10. Top with Romano and serve.
Nutrition Info: Calories: 574, Sodium: 1198 mg, Dietary Fiber: 13.7 g, Total Fat: 14.0 g, Total Carbs: 81.1 g, Protein: 31.1 g.

171.Grandma's Meatballs With Spicy Sauce

Servings: 4
Cooking Time: 20 Minutes
Ingredients:
- 4 tablespoons pork rinds
- 1/3 cup green onion

- 1 pound beef sausage meat
- 3 garlic cloves, minced
- 1/3 teaspoon ground black pepper
- Sea salt, to taste
- For the sauce:
- 2 tablespoons Worcestershire sauce
- 1/3 yellow onion, minced
- Dash of Tabasco sauce
- 1/3 cup tomato paste
- 1 teaspoon cumin powder
- 1/2 tablespoon balsamic vinegar

Directions:

1. Knead all of the above ingredients until everything is well incorporated.
2. Roll into balls and cook in the preheated Air Fryer at 365 degrees for 13 minutes.
3. In the meantime, in a saucepan, cook the ingredients for the sauce until thoroughly warmed. Serve your meatballs with the tomato sauce and enjoy!

Nutrition Info: 360 Calories; 23g Fat; 6g Carbs; 23g Protein; 4g Sugars; 2g Fiber

MEATLESS RECIPES

172.Paprika Cauliflower

Servings: 4
Cooking Time: 20 Minutes
Ingredients:
- 1 large head cauliflower, broken into small florets
- 2 teaspoons smoked paprika
- 1 teaspoon garlic powder
- Salt and freshly ground black pepper, to taste
- Cooking spray

Directions:
1. Spray the air fryer basket with cooking spray.
2. In a medium bowl, toss the cauliflower florets with the smoked paprika and garlic powder until evenly coated. Sprinkle with salt and pepper.
3. Place the cauliflower florets in the basket and lightly mist with cooking spray.
4. Put the air fryer basket on the baking pan and slide into Rack Position 2, select Air Fry, set temperature to 400ºF (205ºC), and set time to 20 minutes.
5. Stir the cauliflower four times during cooking.
6. Remove the cauliflower from the oven and serve hot.

173.Pineapple Spicy Lemon Kebab

Ingredients:
- 4 tbsp. chopped coriander
- 3 tbsp. cream
- 3 tbsp. chopped capsicum
- 3 eggs
- 2 ½ tbsp. white sesame seeds
- 2 cups cubed pineapples
- 3 onions chopped
- 5 green chilies-roughly chopped
- 1 ½ tbsp. ginger paste
- 1 ½ tsp. garlic paste
- 1 ½ tsp. salt
- 3 tsp. lemon juice
- 2 tsp. garam masala

Directions:
1. Grind the ingredients except for the egg and form a smooth paste. Coat the pineapples in the paste. Now, beat the eggs and add a little salt to it.
2. Dip the coated vegetables in the egg mixture and then transfer to the sesame seeds and coat the pineapples well. Place the vegetables on a stick.
3. Pre heat the oven at 160 degrees Fahrenheit for around 5 minutes. Place the sticks in the basket and let them cook for another 25 minutes at the same temperature. Turn the sticks over in between the cooking process to get a uniform cook.

174.Cashew Cauliflower With Yogurt Sauce

Servings: 2
Cooking Time: 12 Minutes
Ingredients:
- 4 cups cauliflower florets (about half a large head)
- 1 tablespoon olive oil
- 1 teaspoon curry powder
- Salt, to taste
- ½ cup toasted, chopped cashews, for garnish
- Yogurt Sauce:
- ¼ cup plain yogurt
- 2 tablespoons sour cream
- 1 teaspoon honey
- 1 teaspoon lemon juice
- Pinch cayenne pepper
- Salt, to taste
- 1 tablespoon chopped fresh cilantro, plus leaves for garnish

Directions:
1. In a large mixing bowl, toss the cauliflower florets with the olive oil, curry powder, and salt.
2. Place the cauliflower florets in the air fryer basket.
3. Put the air fryer basket on the baking pan and slide into Rack Position 2, select Air Fry, set temperature to 400ºF (205ºC) and set time to 12 minutes.
4. Stir the cauliflower florets twice during cooking.
5. When cooking is complete, the cauliflower should be golden brown.
6. Meanwhile, mix all the ingredients for the yogurt sauce in a small bowl and whisk to combine.
7. Remove the cauliflower from the oven and drizzle with the yogurt sauce. Scatter the toasted cashews and cilantro on top and serve immediately.

175.Garlic Toast With Cheese

Ingredients:
- ¾ cup grated cheese
- 2 tsp. of oregano seasoning
- Some red chili flakes to sprinkle on top
- Take some French bread and cut it into slices
- 1 tbsp. olive oil (Optional)
- 2 tbsp. softened butter
- 4-5 flakes crushed garlic
- A pinch of salt to taste
- ½ tsp. black pepper powder

Directions:

1. Take a clean and dry container. Place all the ingredients mentioned under the heading "Garlic Butter" into it and mix properly to obtain garlic butter. On each slice of the French bread, spread some of this garlic butter. Sprinkle some cheese on top of the layer of butter. Pour some oil if wanted.
2. Sprinkle some chili flakes and some oregano.
3. Pre heat the oven at 240 Fahrenheit for around 5 minutes. Open the fry basket and place the bread in it making sure that no two slices touch each other. Close the basket and continue to cook the bread at 160 degrees for another 10 minutes to toast the bread well.

176.Okra Flat Cakes

Ingredients:
- 2 or 3 green chilies finely chopped
- 1 ½ tbsp. lemon juice
- Salt and pepper to taste
- 2 tbsp. garam masala
- 2 cups sliced okra
- 3 tsp. ginger finely chopped
- 1-2 tbsp. fresh coriander leaves

Directions:
1. Mix the ingredients in a clean bowl and add water to it. Make sure that the
2. paste is not too watery but is enough to apply on the okra.
3. Pre heat the oven at 160 degrees Fahrenheit for 5 minutes. Place the French Cuisine Galettes in the fry basket and let them cook for another 25 minutes at the same temperature. Keep rolling them over to get a uniform cook. Serve either with mint sauce or ketchup.

177.Stuffed Mushrooms

Servings: 12
Cooking Time: 8 Minutes
Ingredients:
- 2 Rashers Bacon, Diced
- ½ Onion, Diced
- ½ Bell Pepper, Diced
- 1 Small Carrot, Diced
- 24 Medium Size Mushrooms (Separate the caps & stalks)
- 1 cup Shredded Cheddar Plus Extra for the Top
- ½ cup Sour Cream

Directions:
1. Preparing the Ingredients. Chop the mushrooms stalks finely and fry them up with the bacon, onion, pepper and carrot at 350 ° for 8 minutes.

2. When the veggies are fairly tender, stir in the sour cream & the cheese. Keep on the heat until the cheese has melted and everything is mixed nicely.
3. Now grab the mushroom caps and heap a plop of filling on each one.
4. Place in the fryer basket and top with a little extra cheese.

178.Pizza

Ingredients:
- 2 tomatoes that have been deseeded and chopped
- 1 tbsp. (optional) mushrooms/corns
- 2 tsp. pizza seasoning
- Some cottage cheese that has been cut into small cubes (optional)
- One pizza base
- Grated pizza cheese (mozzarella cheese preferably) for topping
- Use cooking oil for brushing and topping purposes
- ingredients for topping:
- 2 onions chopped
- 2 capsicums chopped

Directions:
1. Put the pizza base in a pre-heated oven for around 5 minutes. (Pre heated to 340 Fahrenheit). Take out the base.
2. Pour some pizza sauce on top of the base at the center. Using a spoon spread the sauce over the base making sure that you leave some gap around the circumference. Grate some mozzarella cheese and sprinkle it over the sauce layer. Take all the vegetables mentioned in the ingredient list above and mix them in a bowl.
3. Add some oil and seasoning. Also add some salt and pepper according to taste. Mix them properly. Put this topping over the layer of cheese on the pizza. Now sprinkle some more grated cheese and pizza seasoning on top of this layer.
4. Pre heat the oven at 250 Fahrenheit for around 5 minutes. Open the fry basket and place the pizza inside. Close the basket and keep the fryer at 170 degrees for another 10 minutes. If you feel that it is undercooked you may put it at the same temperature for another 2 minutes or so.

179.Tortellini With Veggies And Parmesan

Servings: 4
Cooking Time: 16 Minutes
Ingredients:
- 8 ounces (227 g) sugar snap peas, trimmed

- ½ pound (227 g) asparagus, trimmed and cut into 1-inch pieces
- 2 teaspoons kosher salt or 1 teaspoon fine salt, divided
- 1 tablespoon extra-virgin olive oil
- 1½ cups water
- 1 (20-ounce / 340-g) package frozen cheese tortellini
- 2 garlic cloves, minced
- 1 cup heavy (whipping) cream
- 1 cup cherry tomatoes, halved
- ½ cup grated Parmesan cheese
- ¼ cup chopped fresh parsley or basil
- Add the peas and asparagus to a large bowl. Add ½ teaspoon of kosher salt and the olive oil and toss until well coated. Place the veggies in the baking pan.

Directions:
1. Slide the baking pan into Rack Position 1, select Convection Bake, set the temperature to 450ºF (235ºC), and set the time for 4 minutes.
2. Meanwhile, dissolve 1 teaspoon of kosher salt in the water.
3. Once cooking is complete, remove the pan from the oven and place the tortellini in the pan. Pour the salted water over the tortellini. Put the pan back to the oven.
4. Slide the baking pan into Rack Position 1, select Convection Bake, set temperature to 450ºF (235ºC), and set time for 7 minutes.
5. Meantime, stir together the garlic, heavy cream, and remaining ½ teaspoon of kosher salt in a small bowl.
6. Once cooking is complete, remove the pan from the oven. Blot off any remaining water with a paper towel. Gently stir the ingredients. Drizzle the cream over and top with the tomatoes.
7. Slide the baking pan into Rack Position 2, select Roast, set the temperature to 375ºF (190ºC), and set the time for 5 minutes.
8. After 4 minutes, remove from the oven.
9. Add the Parmesan cheese and stir until the cheese is melted
10. Serve topped with the parsley.

180.Garlicky Veggie Bake

Servings: 3
Cooking Time: 25 Minutes
Ingredients:
- 3 turnips, sliced
- 1 large red onion, cut into rings
- 1 large zucchini, sliced
- Salt and black pepper to taste
- 2 cloves garlic, crushed
- 1 bay leaf, cut in 6 pieces
- 1 tbsp olive oil

Directions:
1. Place the turnips, onion, and zucchini in a bowl. Toss with olive oil, salt, and pepper.
2. Preheat on Air Fry function to 380 F. Place the veggies into a baking pan. Slip the bay leaves in the different parts of the slices and tuck the garlic cloves in between the slices. Cook for 15 minutes. Serve warm with as a side to a meat dish or salad.

181.Veg Momo's Recipe

Ingredients:
- 2 tsp. ginger-garlic paste
- 2 tsp. soya sauce
- 2 tsp. vinegar
- 1 ½ cup all-purpose flour
- ½ tsp. salt or to taste
- 5 tbsp. water
- 2 cup carrots grated
- 2 cup cabbage grated
- 2 tbsp. oil

Directions:
1. Squeeze the dough and cover it with plastic wrap and set aside. Next, cook the ingredients for the filling and try to ensure that the vegetables are covered well with the sauce.
2. Roll the dough and cut it into a square. Place the filling in the center. Now, wrap the dough to cover the filling and pinch the edges together.
3. Pre heat the oven at 200° F for 5 minutes. Place the gnocchi's in the fry basket and close it. Let them cook at the same temperature for another 20 minutes. Recommended sides are chili sauce or ketchup.

182.Onion French Cuisine Galette

Ingredients:
- 2 or 3 green chilies finely chopped
- 1 ½ tbsp. lemon juice
- Salt and pepper to taste
- 2 tbsp. garam masala
- 2 medium onions (Cut long)
- 1 ½ cup coarsely crushed peanuts
- 3 tsp. ginger finely chopped
- 1-2 tbsp. fresh coriander leaves

Directions:
1. Mix the ingredients in a clean bowl.
2. Mold this mixture into round and flat French Cuisine Galettes.
3. Wet the French Cuisine Galettes slightly with water. Coat each French Cuisine Galette with the crushed peanuts.
4. Pre heat the oven at 160 degrees Fahrenheit for 5 minutes. Place the French Cuisine Galettes in the

fry basket and let them cook for another 25 minutes at the same temperature. Keep rolling them over to get a uniform cook. Serve either with mint sauce or ketchup.

183.Cheese And Garlic French Fries

Ingredients:
- 1 cup molten cheese
- 2 tsp. garlic powder
- 1 tbsp. lemon juice
- 2 medium sized potatoes peeled and cut into thick pieces lengthwise
- ingredients for the marinade:
- 1 tbsp. olive oil
- 1 tsp. mixed herbs
- ½ tsp. red chili flakes
- A pinch of salt to taste

Directions:
1. Boil the potatoes and blanch them. Cut the potato into Oregano Fingers. Mix the ingredients for the marinade and add the potato Oregano Fingers to it making sure that they are coated well.
2. Pre heat the oven for around 5 minutes at 300 Fahrenheit. Take out the basket of the fryer and place the potato Oregano Fingers in them. Close the basket.
3. Now keep the fryer at 200 Fahrenheit for 20 or 25 minutes. In between the process, toss the fries twice or thrice so that they get cooked properly.

184.Awesome Sweet Potato Fries

Servings: 4
Cooking Time: 30 Minutes
Ingredients:
- ½ tsp salt
- ½ tsp garlic powder
- ½ tsp chili powder
- ¼ tsp cumin
- 3 tbsp olive oil
- 3 sweet potatoes, cut into thick strips

Directions:
1. In a bowl, mix salt, garlic powder, chili, and cumin, and olive oil. Coat the strips well in this mixture and arrange them in the basket without overcrowding. Fit in the baking tray and cook for 20 minutes at 380 F on Air Fry function or until crispy. Serve.

185.Cinnamon Celery Roots

Servings: 4
Cooking Time: 20 Minutes
Ingredients:
- 2 celery roots, peeled and diced

- 1 teaspoon extra-virgin olive oil
- 1 teaspoon butter, melted
- ½ teaspoon ground cinnamon
- Sea salt and freshly ground black pepper, to taste

Directions:
1. Line the baking pan with aluminum foil.
2. Toss the celery roots with the olive oil in a large bowl until well coated. Transfer them to the prepared baking pan.
3. Slide the baking pan into Rack Position 2, select Roast, set temperature to 350ºF (180ºC), and set time to 20 minutes.
4. When done, the celery roots should be very tender. Remove from the oven to a serving bowl. Stir in the butter and cinnamon and mash them with a potato masher until fluffy.
5. Season with salt and pepper to taste. Serve immediately.

186.Teriyaki Tofu

Servings: 3
Cooking Time: 15 Minutes
Ingredients:
- Nonstick cooking spray
- 14 oz. firm or extra firm tofu, pressed & cut in 1-inch cubes
- ¼ cup cornstarch
- ½ tsp salt
- ½ tsp ginger
- ½ tsp white pepper
- 3 tbsp. olive oil
- 12 oz. bottle vegan teriyaki sauce

Directions:
1. Lightly spray baking pan with cooking spray.
2. In a shallow dish, combine cornstarch, salt, ginger, and pepper.
3. Heat oil in a large skillet over med-high heat.
4. Toss tofu cubes in cornstarch mixture then add to skillet. Cook 5 minutes, turning over halfway through, until tofu is nicely seared. Transfer the tofu to the prepared baking pan.
5. Set oven to convection bake on 350°F for 15 minutes.
6. Pour all but ½ cup teriyaki sauce over tofu and stir to coat. After oven has preheated for 5 minutes, place the baking pan in position 2 and bake tofu 10 minutes.
7. Turn tofu over, spoon the sauce in the pan over it and bake another 10 minutes. Serve with reserved sauce for dipping.
Nutrition Info: Calories 469, Total Fat 25g, Saturated Fat 4g, Total Carbs 33g, Net Carbs 30g, Protein 28g, Sugar 16g, Fiber 3g, Sodium 2424mg, Potassium 571mg, Phosphorus 428mg

187.Cayenne Spicy Green Beans

Servings: 4
Cooking Time: 20 Minutes
Ingredients:
- 1 cup panko breadcrumbs
- 2 whole eggs, beaten
- ½ cup Parmesan cheese, grated
- ½ cup flour
- 1 tsp cayenne pepper
- 1 ½ pounds green beans
- Salt to taste

Directions:
1.   In a bowl, mix panko breadcrumbs, Parmesan cheese, cayenne pepper, salt, and pepper. Roll the green beans in flour and dip in eggs. Dredge beans in the parmesan-panko mix. Place the prepared beans in the greased cooking basket and fit in the baking tray; cook for 15 minutes on Air Fry function at 350 F, shaking once. Serve and enjoy!

188.Aloo Marinade Cutlet

Ingredients:
- 4 tsp. fennel
- 2 tbsp. ginger-garlic paste
- 1 small onion
- 6-7 flakes garlic (optional)
- Salt to taste
- 4 medium potatoes (cut them into cubes)
- 1 big capsicum (Cut this capsicum into big cubes)
- 1 onion (Cut it into quarters. Now separate the layers carefully.)
- 5 tbsp. gram flour
- A pinch of salt to taste
- 2 cup fresh green coriander
- ½ cup mint leaves
- 3 tbsp. lemon juice

Directions:
1.   Take a clean and dry container. Put into it the coriander, mint, fennel, and ginger, onion/garlic, salt and lemon juice. Mix them.
2.   Pour the mixture into a grinder and blend until you get a thick paste. Now move on to the potato pieces. Slit these pieces almost till the end and leave them aside. Now stuff all the pieces with the paste that was obtained from the previous step. Now leave the stuffed potato aside. Take the sauce and add to it the gram flour and some salt. Mix them together properly. Rub this mixture all over the stuffed potato pieces.
3.   Now leave the cottage cheese aside. Now, to the leftover sauce, add the capsicum and onions. Apply the sauce generously on each of the pieces of capsicum and onion. Now take satay sticks and arrange the potato pieces and vegetables on separate sticks. Pre heat the oven at 290 Fahrenheit for around 5 minutes.
4.   Open the basket. Arrange the satay sticks properly. Close the basket. Keep the sticks with the cottage cheese at 180 degrees for around half an hour while the sticks with the vegetables are to be kept at the same temperature for only 7 minutes. Turn the sticks in between so that one side does not get burnt and also to provide a uniform cook.

189.Apricot Spicy Lemon Kebab

Ingredients:
- 3 tsp. lemon juice
- 2 tsp. garam masala
- 3 eggs
- 2 ½ tbsp. white sesame seeds
- 2 cups fresh apricots
- 3 onions chopped
- 5 green chilies-roughly chopped
- 1 ½ tbsp. ginger paste
- 1 ½ tsp. garlic paste
- 1 ½ tsp. salt

Directions:
1.   Grind the ingredients except for the egg and form a smooth paste. Coat the apricots in the paste. Now, beat the eggs and add a little salt to it.
2.   Dip the coated apricots in the egg mixture and then transfer to the sesame seeds and coat the apricots well. Place the vegetables on a stick.
3.   Pre heat the oven at 160 degrees Fahrenheit for around 5 minutes. Place the sticks in the basket and let them cook for another 25 minutes at the same temperature. Turn the sticks over in between the cooking process to get a uniform cook.

190.Okra Spicy Lemon Kebab

Ingredients:
- 3 tsp. lemon juice
- 2 tsp. garam masala
- 4 tbsp. chopped coriander
- 3 tbsp. cream
- 3 tbsp. chopped capsicum
- 3 eggs
- 2 cups sliced okra
- 3 onions chopped
- 5 green chilies-roughly chopped
- 1 ½ tbsp. ginger paste
- 1 ½ tsp. garlic paste
- 1 ½ tsp. salt
- 2 ½ tbsp. white sesame seeds

Directions:

1. Grind the ingredients except for the egg and form a smooth paste. Coat the okra in the paste. Now, beat the eggs and add a little salt to it.
2. Dip the coated vegetables in the egg mixture and then transfer to the sesame seeds and coat the okra well. Place the vegetables on a stick.
3. Pre heat the oven at 160 degrees Fahrenheit for around 5 minutes. Place the sticks in the basket and let them cook for another 25 minutes at the same temperature. Turn the sticks over in between the cooking process to get a uniform cook.

191.Roasted Bell Peppers With Garlic

Servings: 4
Cooking Time: 22 Minutes
Ingredients:
- 1 green bell pepper, sliced into 1-inch strips
- 1 red bell pepper, sliced into 1-inch strips
- 1 orange bell pepper, sliced into 1-inch strips
- 1 yellow bell pepper, sliced into 1-inch strips
- 2 tablespoons olive oil, divided
- ½ teaspoon dried marjoram
- Pinch salt
- Freshly ground black pepper, to taste
- 1 head garlic

Directions:
1. Toss the bell peppers with 1 tablespoon of olive oil in a large bowl until well coated. Season with the marjoram, salt, and pepper. Toss again and set aside.
2. Cut off the top of a head of garlic. Place the garlic cloves on a large square of aluminum foil. Drizzle the top with the remaining 1 tablespoon of olive oil and wrap the garlic cloves in foil.
3. Transfer the garlic to the air fryer basket.
4. Put the air fryer basket on the baking pan and slide into Rack Position 2, select Roast, set temperature to 330ºF (166ºC) and set time to 15 minutes.
5. After 15 minutes, remove from the oven and add the bell peppers. Return to the oven and set time to 7 minutes.
6. When cooking is complete or until the garlic is soft and the bell peppers are tender.
7. Transfer the cooked bell peppers to a plate. Remove the garlic and unwrap the foil. Let the garlic rest for a few minutes. Once cooled, squeeze the roasted garlic cloves out of their skins and add them to the plate of bell peppers. Stir well and serve immediately.

192.Nutmeg Broccoli With Eggs & Cheddar Cheese

Servings: 4

Cooking Time: 15 Minutes
Ingredients:
- 1 lb broccoli, cut into florets
- 4 eggs
- 1 cup cheddar cheese, shredded
- 1 cup heavy cream
- 1 pinch of nutmeg
- 1 tsp ginger powder

Directions:
1. In boiling water, steam the broccoli for 5 minutes. Drain and place in a bowl. Add in 1 egg, heavy cream, nutmeg, and ginger. Divide the mixture between greased ramekins and sprinkle the cheddar cheese on top. Cook for 10 minutes at 280 F on AirFry function.

193.Cottage Cheese And Mushroom Mexican Burritos

Ingredients:
- ½ cup mushrooms thinly sliced
- 1 cup cottage cheese cut in too long and slightly thick Oregano Fingers
- A pinch of salt to taste
- ½ tsp. red chili flakes
- 1 tsp. freshly ground peppercorns
- ½ cup pickled jalapenos
- 1-2 lettuce leaves shredded.
- ½ cup red kidney beans (soaked overnight)
- ½ small onion chopped
- 1 tbsp. olive oil
- 2 tbsp. tomato puree
- ¼ tsp. red chili powder
- 1 tsp. of salt to taste
- 4-5 flour tortillas
- 1 or 2 spring onions chopped finely. Also cut the greens.
- Take one tomato. Remove the seeds and chop it into small pieces.
- 1 green chili chopped.
- 1 cup of cheddar cheese grated.
- 1 cup boiled rice (not necessary).
- A few flour tortillas to put the filing in.

Directions:
1. Cook the beans along with the onion and garlic and mash them finely.
2. Now, make the sauce you will need for the burrito. Ensure that you create a slightly thick sauce.
3. For the filling, you will need to cook the ingredients well in a pan and ensure that the vegetables have browned on the outside.
4. To make the salad, toss the ingredients together. Place the tortilla and add a layer of sauce, followed by the beans and the filling at the center. Before you

roll it, you will need to place the salad on top of the filling.

5. Pre-heat the oven for around 5 minutes at 200 Fahrenheit. Open the fry basket and keep the burritos inside. Close the basket properly. Let the Air

6. Fryer remain at 200 Fahrenheit for another 15 minutes or so. Halfway through, remove the basket and turn all the burritos over in order to get a uniform cook.

194.White Lentil French Cuisine Galette

Ingredients:
- 1 ½ tbsp. lemon juice
- Salt and pepper to taste
- 2 cup white lentil soaked
- 3 tsp. ginger finely chopped
- 1-2 tbsp. fresh coriander leaves
- 2 or 3 green chilies finely chopped

Directions:
1. Wash the soaked lentils and mix it with the rest of the ingredients in a clean bowl.
2. Mold this mixture into round and flat French Cuisine Galettes.
3. Wet the French Cuisine Galettes slightly with water.
4. Pre heat the oven at 160 degrees Fahrenheit for 5 minutes. Place the French Cuisine Galettes in the fry basket and let them cook for another 25 minutes at the same temperature. Keep rolling them over to get a uniform cook. Serve either with mint sauce or ketchup.

195.Asparagus French Cuisine Galette

Ingredients:
- 1 ½ tbsp. lemon juice
- Salt and pepper to taste
- 2 cups minced asparagus
- 3 tsp. ginger finely chopped
- 1-2 tbsp. fresh coriander leaves
- 2 or 3 green chilies finely chopped

Directions:
1. Mix the ingredients in a clean bowl.
2. Mold this mixture into round and flat French Cuisine Galettes.
3. Wet the French Cuisine Galettes slightly with water.
4. Pre heat the oven at 160 degrees Fahrenheit for 5 minutes. Place the French Cuisine Galettes in the fry basket and let them cook for another 25 minutes at the same temperature. Keep rolling them over to get a uniform cook. Serve either with mint sauce or ketchup.

196.Spaghetti Squash Lasagna

Servings: 4
Cooking Time: 15 Minutes
Ingredients:
- 3 lb. spaghetti squash, halved lengthwise & seeded
- 4 tbsp. water, divided
- 1 tbsp. extra-virgin olive oil
- 1 bunch broccolini, chopped
- 4 cloves garlic, chopped fine
- ¼ tsp crushed red pepper flakes
- 1 cup mozzarella cheese, grated &divided
- ¼ cup parmesan cheese, grated & divided
- ¾ tsp Italian seasoning
- ½ tsp salt
- ¼ tsp ground pepper

Directions:
1. Place squash, cut side down, in a microwave safe dish. Add 2 tablespoons water and microwave on high until tender, about 10 minutes.
2. Heat oil in a large skillet over medium heat. Add broccoli, garlic, and red pepper. Cook, stirring frequently, 2 minutes.
3. Add remaining water and cook until broccolini is tender, about 3-5 minutes. Transfer to a large bowl.
4. With a fork, scrape the squash from the shells into the bowl with the broccolini. Place the shells in an 8x11-inch baking pan.
5. Add ¾ cup mozzarella, 2 tablespoons parmesan, and seasonings to the squash mixture and stir to combine. Spoon evenly into the shells and top with remaining cheese.
6. Place rack in position 1 and set oven to bake on 450°F for 15 minutes. After 5 minutes, place the squash in the oven and cook 10 minutes.
7. Set the oven to broil on high and move the pan to position 2. Broil until cheese starts to brown, about 2 minutes. Serve immediately.

Nutrition Info: Calories 328, Total Fat 6g, Saturated Fat 2g, Total Carbs 48g, Net Carbs 39g, Protein 18g, Sugar 3g, Fiber 9g, Sodium 674mg, Potassium 1714mg, Phosphorus 452mg

197.Easy Cheesy Vegetable Quesadilla

Servings: 1
Cooking Time: 10 Minutes
Ingredients:
- 1 teaspoon olive oil
- 2 flour tortillas
- ¼ zucchini, sliced
- ¼ yellow bell pepper, sliced
- ¼ cup shredded gouda cheese
- 1 tablespoon chopped cilantro
- ½ green onion, sliced

Directions:
1. Coat the air fryer basket with 1 teaspoon of olive oil.
2. Arrange a flour tortilla in the basket and scatter the top with zucchini, bell pepper, gouda cheese, cilantro, and green onion. Place the other flour tortilla on top.
3. Put the air fryer basket on the baking pan and slide into Rack Position 2, select Air Fry, set temperature to 390ºF (199ºC), and set time to 10 minutes.
4. When cooking is complete, the tortillas should be lightly browned and the vegetables should be tender. Remove from the oven and cool for 5 minutes before slicing into wedges.

198.Baked Chickpea Stars

Ingredients:
- 4 tbsp. roasted sesame seeds
- 2 small onion finely chopped
- ½ tsp. coriander powder
- ½ tsp. cumin powder
- Use olive oil for greasing purposes
- 1 cup white chick peas soaked overnight
- 1 tsp. ginger-garlic paste
- 4 tbsp. chopped coriander leaves
- 2 green chilies finely chopped
- 4 tbsp. thick curd
- Pinches of salt and pepper to taste
- 1 tsp. dry mint

Directions:
1. Since the chickpeas have been soaked you will first have to drain them. Add a pinch of salt and pour water until the chickpeas are submerged. Put this container in a pressure cooker and let the chickpeas cook for around 25 minutes until they turn soft. Remove the cooker from the flame. Now mash the chickpeas.
2. Take another container. Into it add the ginger garlic paste, onions, coriander leaves, coriander powder, cumin powder, green chili, salt and pepper, and 1 tbsp. Use your hands to mix these ingredients Pour this mixture into the container with the mashed chickpeas and mix. Spread this mixture over a flat surface to about a half-inch thickness.
3. Cut star shapes out of this layer. Make a mixture of curd and mint leaves and spread this over the surface of the star shaped cutlets. Coat all the sides with sesame seeds. Pre heat the oven at 200-degree Fahrenheit for 5 minutes. Open the basket of the Fryer and put the stars inside. Close the basket properly. Continue to cook the stars for around half an hour. Periodically turn over the stars in the basket in order to prevent overcooking one side. Serve either with mint sauce or tomato ketchup.

199.Roasted Fall Veggies

Servings: 6
Cooking Time: 30 Minutes
Ingredients:
- 2 cups sweet potatoes, cubed
- 2 cups Brussel sprouts, halved
- 3 cups button mushrooms, halved
- ½ red onion, chopped
- 3 cloves garlic, chopped fine
- 4 sage leaves, chopped
- 2 sprigs rosemary, chopped
- 2 sprigs thyme, chopped
- 1 tsp garlic powder
- 1 tsp onion powder
- ½ tsp salt
- ¼ tsp pepper
- 3 tbsp. balsamic vinegar
- Nonstick cooking spray

Directions:
1. Chop vegetables so that they are as close to equal in size as possible. Roughly chop the herbs.
2. In a large bowl, toss vegetables, herbs, and spices to mix. Drizzle vinegar overall and toss to coat.
3. Spray the baking pan with cooking spray. Set oven to bake on 350°F for 35 minutes.
4. Transfer the vegetable mixture to the baking pan and after 5 minutes, place in the oven in position 1. Bake vegetables 25-30 minutes or until vegetables are tender. Turn them over halfway through cooking. Serve immediately.

Nutrition Info: Calories 76, Total Fat 0g, Saturated Fat 0g, Total Carbs 16g, Net Carbs 13g, Protein 3g, Sugar 5g, Fiber 3g, Sodium 231mg, Potassium 455mg, Phosphorus 92mg

200.Cheese Stuffed Green Peppers With Tomato Sauce

Servings: 4
Cooking Time: 35 Minutes
Ingredients:
- 2 cans green chili peppers
- 1 cup cheddar cheese, shredded
- 1 cup Monterey Jack cheese, shredded
- 2 tbsp all-purpose flour
- 2 large eggs, beaten
- ½ cup milk
- 1 can tomato sauce

Directions:
1. Preheat Breville on AirFry function to 380 F. Spray a baking dish with cooking spray. Take half of the chilies and arrange them in the baking dish. Top with half of the cheese and cover with the remaining

chilies. In a medium bowl, combine eggs, milk, and flour and pour over the chilies.

2. Press Start and cook for 20 minutes. Remove the chilies and pour the tomato sauce over them; cook for 15 more minutes. Top with the remaining cheese and serve.

201.Gourd French Cuisine Galette

Ingredients:
- 2 or 3 green chilies finely chopped
- 1 ½ tbsp. lemon juice
- Salt and pepper to taste
- 2 tbsp. garam masala
- 2 cups sliced gourd
- 1 ½ cup coarsely crushed peanuts
- 3 tsp. ginger finely chopped
- 1-2 tbsp. fresh coriander leaves

Directions:
1. Mix the ingredients in a clean bowl.
2. Mold this mixture into round and flat French Cuisine Galettes.
3. Wet the French Cuisine Galettes slightly with water. Coat each French Cuisine Galette with the crushed peanuts.
4. Pre heat the oven at 160 degrees Fahrenheit for 5 minutes. Place the French Cuisine Galettes in the fry basket and let them cook for another 25 minutes at the same temperature. Keep rolling them over to get a uniform cook. Serve either with mint sauce or ketchup

202.Chickpea Fritters

Servings: 4
Cooking Time: 10 Minutes
Ingredients:
- Nonstick cooking spray
- 1 cup chickpeas, cooked
- 1 onion, chopped
- ¼ tsp salt
- ¼ tsp pepper
- ¼ tsp turmeric
- ¼ tsp coriander

Directions:
1. Place the baking pan in position 2. Lightly spray the fryer basket with cooking spray.
2. Add the onion to a food processor and pulse until finely diced.
3. Add remaining ingredients and pulse until combined but not pureed.
4. Form the mixture into 8 patties and place them in the fryer basket, these may need to be cooked in two batches.

5. Place the basket in the oven and set to air fry on 350°F for 10 minutes. Cook fritters until golden brown and crispy, turning over halfway through cooking time. Serve with your favorite dipping sauce.
Nutrition Info: Calories 101, Total Fat 1g, Saturated Fat 0g, Total Carbs 14g, Net Carbs 10g, Protein 4g, Sugar 3g, Fiber 4g, Sodium 149mg, Potassium 159mg, Phosphorus 77mg

203.Cottage Cheese Flat Cakes

Ingredients:
- 2 or 3 green chilies finely chopped
- 1 ½ tbsp. lemon juice
- Salt and pepper to taste
- 2 tbsp. garam masala
- 2 cups sliced cottage cheese
- 3 tsp. ginger finely chopped
- 1-2 tbsp. fresh coriander leaves

Directions:
1. Mix the ingredients in a clean bowl and add water to it. Make sure that the paste is not too watery but is enough to apply on the cottage cheese slices.
2. Pre heat the oven at 160 degrees Fahrenheit for 5 minutes. Place the French Cuisine Galettes in the fry basket and let them cook for another 25 minutes at the same temperature. Keep rolling them over to get a uniform cook. Serve either with mint sauce or ketchup.

204.Cottage Cheese Gnocchi's

Ingredients:
- 2 tsp. ginger-garlic paste
- 2 tsp. soya sauce
- 2 tsp. vinegar
- 1 ½ cup all-purpose flour
- ½ tsp. salt
- 5 tbsp. water
- 2 cups grated cottage cheese
- 2 tbsp. oil

Directions:
1. Squeeze the dough and cover it with plastic wrap and set aside. Next, cook the ingredients for the filling and try to ensure that the cottage cheese is covered well with the sauce.
2. Roll the dough and place the filling in the center. Now, wrap the dough to cover the filling and pinch the edges together.
3. Pre heat the oven at 200° F for 5 minutes. Place the gnocchi's in the fry basket and close it. Let them cook at the same temperature for another 20 minutes. Recommended sides are chili sauce or ketchup.

205.Roasted Vegetable Mélange With Herbs

Servings: 4
Cooking Time: 16 Minutes
Ingredients:
- 1 (8-ounce / 227-g) package sliced mushrooms
- 1 yellow summer squash, sliced
- 1 red bell pepper, sliced
- 3 cloves garlic, sliced
- 1 tablespoon olive oil
- ½ teaspoon dried basil
- ½ teaspoon dried thyme
- ½ teaspoon dried tarragon

Directions:
1. Toss the mushrooms, squash, and bell pepper with the garlic and olive oil in a large bowl until well coated. Mix in the basil, thyme, and tarragon and toss again.
2. Spread the vegetables evenly in the air fryer basket.
3. Put the air fryer basket on the baking pan and slide into Rack Position 2, select Roast, set temperature to 350ºF (180ºC), and set time to 16 minutes.
4. When cooking is complete, the vegetables should be fork-tender. Remove from the oven and cool for 5 minutes before serving.

206.Radish Flat Cakes

Ingredients:
- 1-2 tbsp. fresh coriander leaves
- 2 or 3 green chilies finely chopped
- 1 ½ tbsp. lemon juice
- Salt and pepper to taste
- 2 tbsp. garam masala
- 2 cups sliced radish
- 3 tsp. ginger finely chopped

Directions:
1. Mix the ingredients in a clean bowl and add water to it. Make sure that the paste is not too watery but is enough to apply on the radish.
2. Pre heat the oven at 160 degrees Fahrenheit for 5 minutes. Place the French Cuisine Galettes in the fry basket and let them cook for another 25 minutes at the same temperature. Keep rolling them over to get a uniform cook. Serve either with mint sauce or ketchup.

207.Cottage Cheese Fried Baked Pastry

Ingredients:
- 1 or 2 green chilies that are finely chopped or mashed
- ½ tsp. cumin
- 1 tsp. coarsely crushed coriander
- 1 dry red chili broken into pieces
- A small amount of salt (to taste)
- ½ tsp. dried mango powder
- ½ tsp. red chili power
- 1-2 tbsp. coriander
- 2 tbsp. unsalted butter
- 1 ½ cup all-purpose flour
- A pinch of salt to taste
- Water
- 2 cups mashed cottage cheese
- ¼ cup boiled peas
- 1 tsp. powdered ginger

Directions:
1. Mix the dough for the outer covering and make it stiff and smooth. Leave it to rest in a container while making the filling.
2. Cook the ingredients in a pan and stir them well to make a thick paste. Roll the paste out.
3. Roll the dough into balls and flatten them. Cut them in halves and add the filling. Use water to help you fold the edges to create the shape of a cone.
4. Pre-heat the oven for around 5 to 6 minutes at 300 Fahrenheit. Place all the samosas in the fry basket and close the basket properly. Keep the oven at 200 degrees for another 20 to 25 minutes. Around the halfway point, open the basket and turn the samosas over for uniform cooking. After this, fry at 250 degrees for around 10 minutes in order to give them the desired golden-brown color. Serve hot. Recommended sides are tamarind or mint sauce.

208.Garlic Stuffed Mushrooms

Servings: 2
Cooking Time: 12 Minutes
Ingredients:
- 18 medium-sized white mushrooms
- 1 small onion, peeled and chopped
- 4 garlic cloves, peeled and minced
- 2 tablespoons olive oil
- 2 teaspoons cumin powder
- A pinch ground allspice
- Fine sea salt and freshly ground black pepper, to taste

Directions:
1. On a clean work surface, remove the mushroom stems. Using a spoon, scoop out the mushroom gills and discard.
2. Thoroughly combine the onion, garlic, olive oil, cumin powder, allspice, salt, and pepper in a mixing bowl. Stuff the mushrooms evenly with the mixture.
3. Place the stuffed mushrooms in the air fryer basket.

4. Put the air fryer basket on the baking pan and slide into Rack Position 2, select Roast, set temperature to 345ºF (174ºC) and set time to 12 minutes.
5. When cooking is complete, the mushroom should be browned.
6. Cool for 5 minutes before serving.

209.Crispy Fried Okra With Chili

Servings: 4
Cooking Time: 10 Minutes
Ingredients:
- 3 tablespoons sour cream
- 2 tablespoons flour
- 2 tablespoons semolina
- ½ teaspoon red chili powder
- Salt and black pepper, to taste
- 1 pound (454 g) okra, halved
- Cooking spray

Directions:
1. Spray the air fryer basket with cooking spray. Set aside.
2. In a shallow bowl, place the sour cream. In another shallow bowl, thoroughly combine the flour, semolina, red chili powder, salt, and pepper.
3. Dredge the okra in the sour cream, then roll in the flour mixture until evenly coated. Transfer the okra to the air fryer basket.
4. Put the air fryer basket on the baking pan and slide into Rack Position 2, select Air Fry, set temperature to 400ºF (205ºC), and set time to 10 minutes.
5. Flip the okra halfway through the cooking time.
6. When cooking is complete, the okra should be golden brown and crispy. Remove from the oven and cool for 5 minutes before serving.

210.Herby Tofu

Servings: 2
Cooking Time: 30 Minutes
Ingredients:
- 6 oz extra firm tofu
- Black pepper to taste
- 1 tbsp vegetable broth
- 1 tbsp soy sauce
- ⅓ tsp dried oregano
- ⅓ tsp garlic powder
- ⅓ tsp dried basil
- ⅓ tsp onion powder

Directions:
1. Place the tofu on a cutting board and cut it into 3 lengthwise slices with a knife. Line a side of the cutting board with paper towels, place the tofu on it, and cover with a paper towel. Use your hands to press the tofu gently until as much liquid has been extracted from it. Chop the tofu into 8 cubes; set aside.
2. In another bowl, add the soy sauce, vegetable broth, oregano, basil, garlic powder, onion powder, and black pepper and mix well with a spoon. Rub the spice mixture on the tofu. Let it marinate for 10 minutes.
3. Preheat on Air Fry function to 390 F. Place the tofu in the fryer's basket in a single layer and fit in the baking tray. Cook for 10 minutes, flipping it at the 6-minute mark. Remove to a plate and serve with green salad.

211.Banana Best Homemade Croquette

Ingredients:
- 2 tsp. garam masala
- 4 tbsp. chopped coriander
- 3 tbsp. cream
- 3 tbsp. chopped capsicum
- 3 eggs
- 2 ½ tbsp. white sesame seeds
- 2 cups sliced banana
- 3 onions chopped
- 5 green chilies-roughly chopped
- 1 ½ tbsp. ginger paste
- 1 ½ tsp. garlic paste
- 1 ½ tsp. salt
- 3 tsp. lemon juice

Directions:
1. Grind the ingredients except for the egg and form a smooth paste. Coat the banana in the paste. Now, beat the eggs and add a little salt to it.
2. Dip the coated bananas in the egg mixture and then transfer to the sesame seeds and coat the vegetables well. Place the vegetables on a stick.
3. Pre heat the oven at 160 degrees Fahrenheit for around 5 minutes. Place the sticks in the basket and let them cook for another 25 minutes at the same temperature. Turn the sticks over in between the cooking process to get a uniform cook.

212.Tomato & Feta Bites With Pine Nuts

Servings: 2
Cooking Time: 25 Minutes
Ingredients:
- 1 heirloom tomato, sliced
- 1 (4- oz) block Feta cheese, sliced
- 1 small red onion, thinly sliced
- 1 clove garlic
- 2 tsp + ¼ cup olive oil
- 1 ½ tbsp toasted pine nuts

- ¼ cup fresh parsley, chopped
- ¼ cup grated Parmesan cheese
- ¼ cup chopped basil

Directions:

1.   Add basil, pine nuts, garlic, and salt to a food processor. Process while slowly adding ¼ cup of olive oil. Once finished, pour basil pesto into a bowl and refrigerate for 30 minutes.

2.   Preheat Breville oven on AirFry function to 390 F. Spread some pesto on each slice of tomato.

3.   Top with feta cheese and onion and drizzle with the remaining olive oil. Place in the frying basket and press Start. Cook for 12 minutes. Top with the remaining pesto and serve.

213.Macaroni Fried Baked Pastry

Ingredients:

- 2 carrot sliced
- 2 cabbage sliced
- 2 tbsp. soya sauce
- 2 tsp. vinegar
- Some salt and pepper to taste
- 2 tbsp. olive oil
- ½ tsp. axiomata
- 1 cup all-purpose flour
- 2 tbsp. unsalted butter
- A pinch of salt to taste
- Take the amount of water sufficient enough to make a stiff dough
- 3 cups boiled macaroni
- 2 onion sliced
- 2 capsicum sliced
- 2 tbsp. ginger finely chopped
- 2 tbsp. garlic finely chopped
- 2 tbsp. green chilies finely chopped
- 2 tbsp. ginger-garlic paste

Directions:

1.   Mix the dough for the outer covering and make it stiff and smooth. Leave it to rest in a container while making the filling. Cook the ingredients in a pan and stir them well to make a thick paste. Roll the paste out.

2.   Roll the dough into balls and flatten them. Cut them in halves and add the filling. Use water to help you fold the edges to create the shape of a cone. Preheat the oven for around 5 to 6 minutes at 300 Fahrenheit. Place all the samosas in the fry basket and close the basket properly. Keep the oven at 200 degrees for another 20 to 25 minutes.

3.   Around the halfway point, open the basket and turn the samosas over for uniform cooking. After this, fry at 250 degrees for around 10 minutes in order to give them the desired golden-brown color. Serve hot. Recommended sides are tamarind or mint sauce.

214.Cheese And Mushroom Spicy Lemon Kebab

Ingredients:

- 1-2 tbsp. all-purpose flour for coating purposes
- 1-2 tbsp. mint
- 1 cup molten cheese
- 1 onion that has been finely chopped
- ½ cup milk
- 2 cups sliced mushrooms
- 1-2 green chilies chopped finely
- ¼ tsp. red chili powder
- A pinch of salt to taste
- ½ tsp. dried mango powder
- ¼ tsp. black salt

Directions:

1.   Take the mushroom slices and add the grated ginger and the cut green chilies. Grind this mixture until it becomes a thick paste.

2.   Keep adding water as and when required. Now add the onions, mint, the breadcrumbs and all the various masalas required. Mix this well until you get a soft dough. Now take small balls of this mixture (about the size of a lemon) and mold them into the shape of flat and round kebabs. Here is where the milk comes into play.

3.   Pour a very small amount of milk onto each kebab to wet it. Now roll the kebab in the dry breadcrumbs. Pre heat the oven for 5 minutes at 300 Fahrenheit. Take out the basket. Arrange the kebabs in the basket leaving gaps between them so that no two kebabs are touching each other. Keep the fryer at 340 Fahrenheit for around half an hour.

4.   Half way through the cooking process, turn the kebabs over so that they can be cooked properly. Recommended sides for this dish are mint sauce, tomato ketchup or yoghurt sauce.

215.Eggplant Patties With Mozzarella

Servings: 1
Cooking Time: 10 Minutes
Ingredients:

- 1 hamburger bun
- 2-inch eggplant slices, cut along the round axis
- 1 mozzarella cheese slice
- 3 red onion rings
- 1 lettuce leaf
- ½ tbsp tomato sauce
- 1 pickle, sliced

Directions:

1.   Preheat Breville on Bake function to 330 F. Cook in the eggplant slices to roast for 6 minutes. Place the mozzarella slice on top of the eggplant and cook for

30 more seconds. Spread tomato sauce on one half of the bun.

2. Place the lettuce leaf on top of the sauce. Place the cheesy eggplant on top of the lettuce. Top with onion rings and pickles, and then with the other bun half and enjoy.

216.Roasted Carrots

Servings: 4
Cooking Time: 15 Minutes
Ingredients:
- 20 oz carrots, julienned
- 1 tbsp olive oil
- 1 tsp cumin seeds
- 2 tbsp fresh cilantro, chopped

Directions:
1. In a bowl, mix olive oil, carrots, and cumin seeds; stir to coat. Place the carrots in a baking tray and cook in your on Bake function at 300 F for 10 minutes. Scatter fresh coriander over the carrots and serve.

217.Vegetarian Meatballs

Servings: 3
Cooking Time: 18 Minutes
Ingredients:
- ½ cup grated carrots
- ½ cup sweet onions
- 2 tablespoons olive oil
- 1 cup rolled oats
- ½ cup roasted cashews
- 2 cups cooked chickpeas
- Juice of 1 lemon
- 2 tablespoons soy sauce
- 1 tablespoon flax meal
- 1 teaspoon garlic powder
- 1 teaspoon cumin
- ½ teaspoon turmeric

Directions:
1. Mix the carrots, onions, and olive oil in the baking pan and stir to combine.
2. Slide the baking pan into Rack Position 2, select Roast, set temperature to 350ºF (180ºC) and set time to 6 minutes.
3. Stir the vegetables halfway through.
4. When cooking is complete, the vegetables should be tender.
5. Meanwhile, put the oats and cashews in a food processor or blender and pulse until coarsely ground. Transfer the mixture to a large bowl. Add the chickpeas, lemon juice, and soy sauce to the food processor and pulse until smooth. Transfer the

chickpea mixture to the bowl of oat and cashew mixture.
6. Remove the carrots and onions from the oven to the bowl of chickpea mixture. Add the flax meal, garlic powder, cumin, and turmeric and stir to incorporate.
7. Scoop tablespoon-sized portions of the veggie mixture and roll them into balls with your hands. Transfer the balls to the air fryer basket.
8. Increase the temperature to 370ºF (188ºC) and set time to 12 minutes on Bake. Flip the balls halfway through the cooking time.
9. When cooking is complete, the balls should be golden brown.
10. Serve warm.

218.Broccoli Marinade Cutlet

Ingredients:
- 1 ½ tsp. salt
- 3 tsp. lemon juice
- 2 tsp. garam masala
- 3 eggs
- 2 ½ tbsp. white sesame seeds
- 2 cups broccoli florets
- 3 onions chopped
- 5 green chilies-roughly chopped
- 1 ½ tbsp. ginger paste
- 1 ½ tsp. garlic paste

Directions:
1. Grind the ingredients except for the egg and form a smooth paste. Coat the florets in the paste. Now, beat the eggs and add a little salt to it.
2. Dip the coated florets in the egg mixture and then transfer to the sesame seeds and coat the florets well. Place the vegetables on a stick.
3. Pre heat the oven at 160 degrees Fahrenheit for around 5 minutes. Place the sticks in the basket and let them cook for another 25 minutes at the same temperature. Turn the sticks over in between the cooking process to get a uniform cook.

219.Mushroom Fried Baked Pastry

Ingredients:
- 2 capsicum sliced
- 2 carrot sliced
- 2 cabbage sliced
- 2 tbsp. soya sauce
- 2 tsp. vinegar
- 1 cup all-purpose flour
- 2 tbsp. unsalted butter
- A pinch of salt to taste
- Take the amount of water sufficient enough to make a stiff dough

- 3 cups whole mushrooms
- 2 onion sliced
- 2 tbsp. green chilies finely chopped
- 2 tbsp. ginger-garlic paste
- Some salt and pepper to taste

Directions:
1. Mix the dough for the outer covering and make it stiff and smooth. Leave it to rest in a container while making the filling.
2. Cook the ingredients in a pan and stir them well to make a thick paste. Roll the paste out.
3. Roll the dough into balls and flatten them. Cut them in halves and add the filling. Use water to help you fold the edges to create the shape of a cone.
4. Pre-heat the oven for around 5 to 6 minutes at 300 Fahrenheit. Place all the samosas in the fry basket and close the basket properly. Keep the oven at 200 degrees for another 20 to 25 minutes. Around the halfway point, open the basket and turn the samosas over for uniform cooking. After this, fry at 250 degrees for around 10 minutes in order to give them the desired golden-brown color. Serve hot. Recommended sides are tamarind or mint sauce.

220.Cheesy Cabbage Wedges

Servings: 4
Cooking Time: 25 Minutes
Ingredients:
- ½ head cabbage, cut into wedges
- 2 cups Parmesan cheese, chopped
- 4 tbsp melted butter
- Salt and black pepper to taste
- ½ cup blue cheese sauce

Directions:
1. Brush the cabbage wedges with butter and coat with mozzarella cheese. Place the coated wedges in the greased basket and fit in the baking tray; cook for 20 minutes at 380 F on Air Fry setting. Serve with blue cheese sauce.

221.Baby Spinach & Pumpkin With Nuts & Cheese

Servings: 1
Cooking Time: 30 Minutes
Ingredients:
- ½ small pumpkin
- 2 oz blue cheese, crumbled
- 2 tbsp pine nuts
- 1 tbsp olive oil
- ½ cup baby spinach, packed
- 1 spring onion, sliced
- 1 radish, thinly sliced
- 1 tsp vinegar

Directions:
1. Preheat on Toast function to 330 F. Place the pine nuts in the Air Fryer pan and toast them for 5 minutes; set aside. Peel the pumpkin and chop it into small pieces and toss them with olive oil. Place in the Air Fryer basket and fit in the baking tray. Increase the temperature to 390 F and cook for 20 minutes.
2. Remove the pumpkin to a serving bowl. Add in baby spinach, radish, and spring onion; toss with the vinegar. Stir in the blue cheese and top with the toasted pine nuts to serve.

222.Classic Ratatouille

Servings: 2
Cooking Time: 30 Minutes
Ingredients:
- 1 tbsp olive oil
- 3 roma tomatoes, thinly sliced
- 2 garlic cloves, minced
- 1 zucchini, thinly sliced
- 2 yellow bell peppers, sliced
- 1 tbsp red wine vinegar
- 2 tbsp herbs de Provence
- Salt and black pepper to taste

Directions:
1. Preheat on Air Fry function to 390 F. In a bowl, mix together olive oil, garlic, vinegar, herbs, salt, and pepper. Add in tomatoes, zucchini, and bell peppers and toss to coat.
2. Arrange the vegetables in a baking dish and cook for 15 minutes, shaking occasionally. Let sit for 5 more minutes after the timer goes off. Serve.

223.Cottage Cheese Club Sandwich

Ingredients:
- ¼ tbsp. Worcestershire sauce
- ½ tsp. olive oil
- ½ flake garlic crushed
- ¼ cup chopped onion
- ¼ tbsp. red chili sauce
- 2 slices of white bread
- 1 tbsp. softened butter
- 1 cup sliced cottage cheese
- 1 small capsicum

Directions:
1. Take the slices of bread and remove the edges. Now cut the slices horizontally.
2. Cook the ingredients for the sauce and wait till it thickens. Now, add the cottage cheese to the sauce and stir till it obtains the flavors. Roast the capsicum and peel the skin off. Cut the capsicum into slices. Mix the ingredients together and apply it to the bread slices.

3. Pre-heat the oven for 5 minutes at 300 Fahrenheit. Open the basket of the Fryer and place the prepared Classic Sandwiches in it such that no two Classic Sandwiches are touching each other. Now keep the fryer at 250 degrees for around 15 minutes. Turn the Classic Sandwiches in between the cooking process to cook both slices. Serve the Classic Sandwiches with tomato ketchup or mint sauce.

224.Asparagus Spicy Lemon Kebab

Ingredients:
- 3 tsp. lemon juice
- 2 tsp. garam masala
- 3 eggs
- 2 ½ tbsp. white sesame seeds
- 2 cups sliced asparagus
- 3 onions chopped
- 5 green chilies-roughly chopped
- 1 ½ tbsp. ginger paste
- 1 ½ tsp. garlic paste
- 1 ½ tsp. salt

Directions:
1. Grind the ingredients except for the egg and form a smooth paste. Coat the asparagus in the paste. Now, beat the eggs and add a little salt to it.
2. Dip the coated apricots in the egg mixture and then transfer to the sesame seeds and coat the asparagus. Place the vegetables on a stick.
3. Pre heat the oven at 160 degrees Fahrenheit for around 5 minutes. Place the sticks in the basket and let them cook for another 25 minutes at the same temperature. Turn the sticks over in between the cooking process to get a uniform cook.

225.Carrots & Shallots With Yogurt

Servings: 4
Cooking Time: 25 Minutes
Ingredients:
- 2 tsp olive oil
- 2 shallots, chopped
- 3 carrots, sliced
- Salt to taste
- ¼ cup yogurt
- 2 garlic cloves, minced
- 3 tbsp parsley, chopped

Directions:
1. In a bowl, mix sliced carrots, salt, garlic, shallots, parsley, and yogurt. Sprinkle with oil. Place the veggies in the basket and press Start. Cook for 15 minutes on AirFry function at 370 F. Serve with basil and garlic mayo.

226.Crispy Eggplant Slices With Parsley

Servings: 4
Cooking Time: 12 Minutes
Ingredients:
- 1 cup flour
- 4 eggs
- Salt, to taste
- 2 cups bread crumbs
- 1 teaspoon Italian seasoning
- 2 eggplants, sliced
- 2 garlic cloves, sliced
- 2 tablespoons chopped parsley
- Cooking spray

Directions:
1. Spritz the air fryer basket with cooking spray. Set aside.
2. On a plate, place the flour. In a shallow bowl, whisk the eggs with salt. In another shallow bowl, combine the bread crumbs and Italian seasoning.
3. Dredge the eggplant slices, one at a time, in the flour, then in the whisked eggs, finally in the bread crumb mixture to coat well.
4. Lay the coated eggplant slices in the basket.
5. Put the air fryer basket on the baking pan and slide into Rack Position 2, select Air Fry, set temperature to 390ºF (199ºC), and set time to 12 minutes.
6. Flip the eggplant slices halfway through the cooking time.
7. When cooking is complete, the eggplant slices should be golden brown and crispy. Transfer the eggplant slices to a plate and sprinkle the garlic and parsley on top before serving.

227.Zucchini Fried Baked Pastry

Ingredients:
- 1 or 2 green chilies that are finely chopped or mashed
- ½ tsp. cumin
- 1 tsp. coarsely crushed coriander
- 1 dry red chili broken into pieces
- A small amount of salt (to taste)
- ½ tsp. dried mango powder
- ½ tsp. red chili power.
- 2 tbsp. unsalted butter
- 1 ½ cup all-purpose flour
- A pinch of salt to taste
- Add as much water as required to make the dough stiff and firm
- 3 medium zucchinis (mashed)
- ¼ cup boiled peas
- 1 tsp. powdered ginger
- 1-2 tbsp. coriander.

Directions:

1. Mix the dough for the outer covering and make it stiff and smooth. Leave it to rest in a container while making the filling.
2. Cook the ingredients in a pan and stir them well to make a thick paste. Roll the paste out.
3. Roll the dough into balls and flatten them. Cut them in halves and add the
4. filling. Use water to help you fold the edges to create the shape of a cone.
5. Pre-heat the oven for around 5 to 6 minutes at 300 Fahrenheit. Place all the samosas in the fry basket and close the basket properly. Keep the oven at 200 degrees for another 20 to 25 minutes. Around the halfway point, open the basket and turn the samosas over for uniform cooking. After this, fry at 250 degrees for around 10 minutes in order to give them the desired golden-brown color. Serve hot. Recommended sides are tamarind or mint sauce.

228.Mushroom Pops

Ingredients:
- 1 tsp. dry basil
- 1 tsp. lemon juice
- 1 tsp. red chili flakes
- 1 cup whole mushrooms
- 1 ½ tsp. garlic paste
- Salt and pepper to taste
- 1 tsp. dry oregano

Directions:
1. Add the ingredients into a separate bowl and mix them well to get a consistent mixture.
2. Dip the mushrooms in the above mixture and leave them aside for some time.
3. Pre heat the oven at 180° C for around 5 minutes. Place the coated cottage cheese pieces in the fry basket and close it properly. Let them cook at the same temperature for 20 more minutes. Keep turning them over in the basket so that they are cooked properly. Serve with tomato ketchup.

FISH & SEAFOOD RECIPES

229.Breaded Scallops

Servings: 4
Cooking Time: 7 Minutes
Ingredients:
- 1 egg
- 3 tablespoons flour
- 1 cup bread crumbs
- 1 pound (454 g) fresh scallops
- 2 tablespoons olive oil
- Salt and black pepper, to taste

Directions:
1. In a bowl, lightly beat the egg. Place the flour and bread crumbs into separate shallow dishes.
2. Dredge the scallops in the flour and shake off any excess. Dip the flour-coated scallops in the beaten egg and roll in the bread crumbs.
3. Brush the scallops generously with olive oil and season with salt and pepper, to taste. Transfer the scallops to the air fryer basket.
4. Put the air fryer basket on the baking pan and slide into Rack Position 2, select Air Fry, set temperature to 360ºF (182ºC), and set time to 7 minutes.
5. Flip the scallops halfway through the cooking time.
6. When cooking is complete, the scallops should reach an internal temperature of just 145ºF (63ºC) on a meat thermometer. Remove from the oven. Let the scallops cool for 5 minutes and serve.

230.Parmesan-crusted Hake With Garlic Sauce

Servings: 3
Cooking Time: 10 Minutes
Ingredients:
- Fish:
- 6 tablespoons mayonnaise
- 1 tablespoon fresh lime juice
- 1 teaspoon Dijon mustard
- 1 cup grated Parmesan cheese
- Salt, to taste
- ¼ teaspoon ground black pepper, or more to taste
- 3 hake fillets, patted dry
- Nonstick cooking spray
- Garlic Sauce:
- ¼ cup plain Greek yogurt
- 2 tablespoons olive oil
- 2 cloves garlic, minced
- ½ teaspoon minced tarragon leaves

Directions:

1. Mix the mayo, lime juice, and mustard in a shallow bowl and whisk to combine. In another shallow bowl, stir together the grated Parmesan cheese, salt, and pepper.
2. Dredge each fillet in the mayo mixture, then roll them in the cheese mixture until they are evenly coated on both sides.
3. Spray the air fryer basket with nonstick cooking spray. Place the fillets in the pan.
4. Put the air fryer basket on the baking pan and slide into Rack Position 2, select Air Fry, set temperature to 395ºF (202ºC), and set time to 10 minutes.
5. Flip the fillets halfway through the cooking time.
6. Meanwhile, in a small bowl, whisk all the ingredients for the sauce until well incorporated.
7. When cooking is complete, the fish should flake apart with a fork. Remove the fillets from the oven and serve warm alongside the sauce.

231.Parmesan Fish Fillets

Servings: 4
Cooking Time: 17 Minutes
Ingredients:
- $^1/_3$ cup grated Parmesan cheese
- ½ teaspoon fennel seed
- ½ teaspoon tarragon
- $^1/_3$ teaspoon mixed peppercorns
- 2 eggs, beaten
- 4 (4-ounce / 113-g) fish fillets, halved
- 2 tablespoons dry white wine
- 1 teaspoon seasoned salt

Directions:
1. Place the grated Parmesan cheese, fennel seed, tarragon, and mixed peppercorns in a food processor and pulse for about 20 seconds until well combined. Transfer the cheese mixture to a shallow dish.
2. Place the beaten eggs in another shallow dish.
3. Drizzle the dry white wine over the top of fish fillets. Dredge each fillet in the beaten eggs on both sides, shaking off any excess, then roll them in the cheese mixture until fully coated. Season with the salt.
4. Arrange the fillets in the air fryer basket.
5. Put the air fryer basket on the baking pan and slide into Rack Position 2, select Air Fry, set temperature to 345ºF (174ºC), and set time to 17 minutes.
6. Flip the fillets once halfway through the cooking time.
7. When cooking is complete, the fish should be cooked through no longer translucent. Remove from the oven and cool for 5 minutes before serving.

232. Spicy Lemon Cod

Servings: 2
Cooking Time: 10 Minutes
Ingredients:
- 1 lb cod fillets
- 1/4 tsp chili powder
- 1 tbsp fresh parsley, chopped
- 1 1/2 tbsp olive oil
- 1 tbsp fresh lemon juice
- 1/8 tsp cayenne pepper
- 1/4 tsp salt

Directions:
1. Fit the oven with the rack in position
2. Arrange fish fillets in a baking dish. Drizzle with oil and lemon juice.
3. Sprinkle with chili powder, salt, and cayenne pepper.
4. Set to bake at 400 F for 15 minutes. After 5 minutes place the baking dish in the preheated oven.
5. Garnish with parsley and serve.
Nutrition Info: Calories 276 Fat 12.7 g Carbohydrates 0.5 g Sugar 0.2 g Protein 40.7 g Cholesterol 111 mg

233. Perfect Crab Cakes

Servings: 6
Cooking Time: 30 Minutes
Ingredients:
- 16 oz lump crab meat
- 1/4 cup celery, diced
- 1/4 cup onion, diced
- 1 cup crushed crackers
- 1 tsp old bay seasoning
- 1 tsp brown mustard
- 2/3 cup mashed avocado

Directions:
1. Fit the oven with the rack in position
2. Add all ingredients into the bowl and mix until just combined.
3. Make small patties from mixture and place in parchment-lined baking pan.
4. Set to bake at 350 F for 35 minutes. After 5 minutes place the baking dish in the preheated oven.
5. Serve and enjoy.
Nutrition Info: Calories 84 Fat 7.7 g Carbohydrates 4.6 g Sugar 0.8 g Protein 11.5 g Cholesterol 43 mg

234. Lemony Shrimp

Servings: 4
Cooking Time: 8 Minutes
Ingredients:
- 1 pound (454 g) shrimp, deveined
- 4 tablespoons olive oil
- 1½ tablespoons lemon juice
- 1½ tablespoons fresh parsley, roughly chopped
- 2 cloves garlic, finely minced
- 1 teaspoon crushed red pepper flakes, or more to taste
- Garlic pepper, to taste
- Sea salt flakes, to taste

Directions:
1. Toss all the ingredients in a large bowl until the shrimp are coated on all sides.
2. Arrange the shrimp in the air fryer basket.
3. Put the air fryer basket on the baking pan and slide into Rack Position 2, select Air Fry, set temperature to 385ºF (196ºC), and set time to 8 minutes.
4. When cooking is complete, the shrimp should be pink and cooked through. Remove from the oven and serve warm.

235. Lemon Pepper Tilapia Fillets

Servings: 4
Cooking Time: 15 Minutes
Ingredients:
- 1 lb tilapia fillets
- 1 tbsp Italian seasoning
- 2 tbsp canola oil
- 2 tbsp lemon pepper
- Salt to taste
- 2-3 butter buds

Directions:
1. Preheat your Breville oven to 400 F on Bake function. Drizzle tilapia fillets with canola oil. In a bowl, mix salt, lemon pepper, butter buds, and Italian seasoning; spread on the fish. Place the fillet on a baking tray and press Start. Cook for 10 minutes until tender and crispy. Serve warm.

236. Sweet Cajun Salmon

Servings: 1
Cooking Time: 10 Minutes
Ingredients:
- 1 salmon fillet
- ¼ tsp brown sugar
- Juice of ½ lemon
- 1 tbsp cajun seasoning
- 2 lemon wedges
- 1 tbsp chopped parsley

Directions:
1. Preheat on Bake function to 350 F. Combine sugar and lemon juice; coat the salmon with this mixture. Coat with the Cajun seasoning as well. Place

a parchment paper on a baking tray and cook the fish in your for 10 minutes. Serve with lemon wedges and parsley.

237.Spinach & Tuna Balls With Ricotta

Servings: 4
Cooking Time: 20 Minutes
Ingredients:
- 14 oz store-bought crescent dough
- ½ cup spinach, steamed
- 1 cup ricotta cheese, crumbled
- ¼ tsp garlic powder
- 1 tsp fresh oregano, chopped
- ½ cup canned tuna, drained

Directions:
1. Preheat Breville on AirFry function to 350 F. Roll the dough onto a lightly floured flat surface. Combine the ricotta cheese, spinach, tuna, oregano, salt, and garlic powder together in a bowl.
2. Cut the dough into 4 equal pieces. Divide the mixture between the dough pieces. Make sure to place the filling in the center. Fold the dough and secure with a fork. Place onto a lined baking dish and press Start. Cook for 12 minutes until lightly browned. Serve.

238.Bacon-wrapped Scallops

Servings: 4
Cooking Time: 10 Minutes
Ingredients:
- 8 slices bacon, cut in half
- 16 sea scallops, patted dry
- Cooking spray
- Salt and freshly ground black pepper, to taste
- 16 toothpicks, soaked in water for at least 30 minutes

Directions:
1. On a clean work surface, wrap half of a slice of bacon around each scallop and secure with a toothpick.
2. Lay the bacon-wrapped scallops in the air fryer basket in a single layer.
3. Spritz the scallops with cooking spray and sprinkle the salt and pepper to season.
4. Put the air fryer basket on the baking pan and slide into Rack Position 2, select Air Fry, set temperature to 370ºF (188ºC), and set time to 10 minutes.
5. Flip the scallops halfway through the cooking time.
6. When cooking is complete, the bacon should be cooked through and the scallops should be firm.

Remove the scallops from the oven to a plate Serve warm.

239.Prawn Momo's Recipe

Ingredients:
- 1 ½ cup all-purpose flour
- ½ tsp. salt
- 5 tbsp. water
- For filling:
- 2 cups minced prawn
- 2 tbsp. oil
- 2 tsp. ginger-garlic paste
- 2 tsp. soya sauce
- 2 tsp. vinegar

Directions:
1. Squeeze the dough and cover it with plastic wrap and set aside. Next, cook the ingredients for the filling and try to ensure that the prawn is covered well with the sauce. Roll the dough and cut it into a square.
2. Place the filling in the center. Now, wrap the dough to cover the filling and pinch the edges together. Pre heat the oven at 200° F for 5 minutes. Place the wontons in the fry basket and close it. Let them cook at the same temperature for another 20 minutes. Recommended sides are chili sauce or ketchup.

240.Seafood Spring Rolls

Servings: 4
Cooking Time: 20 Minutes
Ingredients:
- 1 tablespoon olive oil
- 2 teaspoons minced garlic
- 1 cup matchstick cut carrots
- 2 cups finely sliced cabbage
- 2 (4-ounce / 113-g) cans tiny shrimp, drained
- 4 teaspoons soy sauce
- Salt and freshly ground black pepper, to taste
- 16 square spring roll wrappers
- Cooking spray

Directions:
1. Spray the air fryer basket with cooking spray. Set aside.
2. Heat the olive oil in a medium skillet over medium heat until it shimmers.
3. Add the garlic to the skillet and cook for 30 seconds. Stir in the cabbage and carrots and sauté for about 5 minutes, stirring occasionally, or until the vegetables are lightly tender.
4. Fold in the shrimp and soy sauce and sprinkle with salt and pepper, then stir to combine. Sauté for another 2 minutes, or until the moisture is

evaporated. Remove from the heat and set aside to cool.

5.   Put a spring roll wrapper on a work surface and spoon 1 tablespoon of the shrimp mixture onto the lower end of the wrapper.

6.   Roll the wrapper away from you halfway, and then fold in the right and left sides, like an envelope. Continue to roll to the very end, using a little water to seal the edge. Repeat with the remaining wrappers and filling.

7.   Place the spring rolls in the air fryer basket in a single layer, leaving space between each spring roll. Mist them lightly with cooking spray.

8.   Put the air fryer basket on the baking pan and slide into Rack Position 2, select Air Fry, set temperature to 375ºF (190ºC), and set time to 10 minutes.

9.   Flip the rolls halfway through the cooking time.

10. When cooking is complete, the spring rolls will be heated through and start to brown. If necessary, continue cooking for 5 minutes more. Remove from the oven and cool for a few minutes before serving.

241.Fish Oregano Fingers

Ingredients:
- ½ lb. firm white fish fillet cut into Oregano Fingers
- 1 tbsp. lemon juice
- 2 cups of dry breadcrumbs
- 1 cup oil for frying
- 1 ½ tbsp. ginger-garlic paste
- 3 tbsp. lemon juice
- 2 tsp salt
- 1 ½ tsp pepper powder
- 1 tsp red chili flakes or to taste
- 3 eggs
- 5 tbsp. corn flour
- 2 tsp tomato ketchup

Directions:
1.   Rub a little lemon juice on the Oregano Fingers and set aside. Wash the fish after an hour and pat dry. Make the marinade and transfer the Oregano Fingers into the marinade. Leave them on a plate to dry for fifteen minutes. Now cover the Oregano Fingers with the crumbs and set aside to dry for fifteen minutes.

2.   Pre heat the oven at 160 degrees Fahrenheit for 5 minutes or so. Keep the fish in the fry basket now and close it properly.

3.   Let the Oregano Fingers cook at the same temperature for another 25 minutes. In between the cooking process, toss the fish once in a while to avoid burning the food. Serve either with tomato ketchup or chili sauce. Mint sauce also works well with the fish.

242.Paprika Shrimp

Servings: 4
Cooking Time: 10 Minutes
Ingredients:
- 1 pound (454 g) tiger shrimp
- 2 tablespoons olive oil
- ½ tablespoon old bay seasoning
- ¼ tablespoon smoked paprika
- ¼ teaspoon cayenne pepper
- A pinch of sea salt

Directions:
1.   Toss all the ingredients in a large bowl until the shrimp are evenly coated.

2.   Arrange the shrimp in the air fryer basket.

3.   Put the air fryer basket on the baking pan and slide into Rack Position 2, select Air Fry, set temperature to 380ºF (193ºC), and set time to 10 minutes.

4.   When cooking is complete, the shrimp should be pink and cooked through. Remove from the oven and serve hot.

243.Herbed Salmon With Roasted Asparagus

Servings: 2
Cooking Time: 12 Minutes
Ingredients:
- 2 teaspoons olive oil, plus additional for drizzling
- 2 (5-ounce / 142-g) salmon fillets, with skin
- Salt and freshly ground black pepper, to taste
- 1 bunch asparagus, trimmed
- 1 teaspoon dried tarragon
- 1 teaspoon dried chives
- Fresh lemon wedges, for serving

Directions:
1.   Rub the olive oil all over the salmon fillets. Sprinkle with salt and pepper to taste.

2.   Put the asparagus on the foil-lined baking pan and place the salmon fillets on top, skin-side down.

3.   Slide the baking pan into Rack Position 2, select Roast, set temperature to 425ºF (220ºC), and set time to 12 minutes.

4.   When cooked, the fillets should register 145ºF (63ºC) on an instant-read thermometer. Remove from the oven and cut the salmon fillets in half crosswise, then use a metal spatula to lift flesh from skin and transfer to a serving plate. Discard the skin and drizzle the salmon fillets with additional olive oil. Scatter with the herbs.

5.   Serve the salmon fillets with roasted asparagus spears and lemon wedges on the side.

244.Spicy Halibut

Servings: 4
Cooking Time: 12 Minutes
Ingredients:
- 1 lb halibut fillets
- 1/2 tsp chili powder
- 1/2 tsp smoked paprika
- 1/4 cup olive oil
- 1/4 tsp garlic powder
- Pepper
- Salt

Directions:
1. Fit the oven with the rack in position
2. Place halibut fillets in a baking dish.
3. In a small bowl, mix oil, garlic powder, paprika, pepper, chili powder, and salt.
4. Brush fish fillets with oil mixture.
5. Set to bake at 425 F for 17 minutes. After 5 minutes place the baking dish in the preheated oven.
6. Serve and enjoy.
Nutrition Info: Calories 236 Fat 15.3 g Carbohydrates 0.5 g Sugar 0.1 g Protein 24 g Cholesterol 36 mg

245.Cajun Salmon With Lemon

Servings: 1
Cooking Time: 10 Minutes
Ingredients:
- 1 salmon fillet
- ¼ tsp brown sugar
- Juice of ½ lemon
- 1 tbsp cajun seasoning
- 2 lemon wedges
- 1 tbsp fresh parsley, chopped

Directions:
1. Preheat Breville on Bake function to 350 F. Combine sugar and lemon and coat in the salmon. Sprinkle with the Cajun seasoning as well. Place a parchment paper on a baking tray and press Start. Cook for 14-16 minutes. Serve with lemon wedges and chopped parsley.

246.Prawn Grandma's Easy To Cook Wontons

Ingredients:
- 1 ½ cup all-purpose flour
- ½ tsp. salt
- 5 tbsp. water
- 2 cups minced prawn
- 2 tbsp. oil
- 2 tsp. ginger-garlic paste
- 2 tsp. soya sauce
- 2 tsp. vinegar

Directions:
1. Squeeze the dough and cover it with plastic wrap and set aside. Next, cook the ingredients for the filling and try to ensure that the prawn is covered well with the sauce. Roll the dough and place the filling in the center.
2. Now, wrap the dough to cover the filling and pinch the edges together. Pre heat the oven at 200° F for 5 minutes. Place the wontons in the fry basket and close it. Let them cook at the same temperature for another 20 minutes. Recommended sides are chili sauce or ketchup.

247.Fish Cakes With Mango Relish

Servings: 4
Cooking Time: 10 Minutes
Ingredients:
- 1 lb White Fish Fillets
- 3 Tbsps Ground Coconut
- 1 Ripened Mango
- ½ Tsps Chili Paste
- Tbsps Fresh Parsley
- 1 Green Onion
- 1 Lime
- 1 Tsp Salt
- 1 Egg

Directions:
1. Preparing the Ingredients. To make the relish, peel and dice the mango into cubes. Combine with a half teaspoon of chili paste, a tablespoon of parsley, and the zest and juice of half a lime.
2. In a food processor, pulse the fish until it forms a smooth texture. Place into a bowl and add the salt, egg, chopped green onion, parsley, two tablespoons of the coconut, and the remainder of the chili paste and lime zest and juice. Combine well
3. Portion the mixture into 10 equal balls and flatten them into small patties. Pour the reserved tablespoon of coconut onto a dish and roll the patties over to coat.
4. Preheat the Air fryer oven to 390 degrees
5. Air Frying. Place the fish cakes into the air fryer oven and cook for 8 minutes. They should be crisp and lightly browned when ready
6. Serve hot with mango relish

248.Dill Salmon Patties

Servings: 2
Cooking Time: 10 Minutes
Ingredients:
- 14 oz can salmon, drained and discard bones
- 1 tsp dill, chopped

- 1 egg, lightly beaten
- 1/4 tsp garlic powder
- 1/2 cup breadcrumbs
- 1/4 cup onion, diced
- Pepper
- Salt

Directions:
1. Fit the oven with the rack in position 2.
2. Add all ingredients into the large bowl and mix well.
3. Make equal shapes of patties from mixture and place in the air fryer basket then place the air fryer basket in the baking pan.
4. Place a baking pan on the oven rack. Set to air fry at 370 F for 10 minutes.
5. Serve and enjoy.

Nutrition Info: Calories 422 Fat 15.7 g Carbohydrates 21.5 g Sugar 2.5 g Protein 46 g Cholesterol 191 mg

249.Easy Shrimp And Vegetable Paella

Servings: 4
Cooking Time: 16 Minutes
Ingredients:
- 1 (10-ounce / 284-g) package frozen cooked rice, thawed
- 1 (6-ounce / 170-g) jar artichoke hearts, drained and chopped
- ¼ cup vegetable broth
- ½ teaspoon dried thyme
- ½ teaspoon turmeric
- 1 cup frozen cooked small shrimp
- ½ cup frozen baby peas
- 1 tomato, diced

Directions:
1. Mix together the cooked rice, chopped artichoke hearts, vegetable broth, thyme, and turmeric in the baking pan and stir to combine.
2. Slide the baking pan into Rack Position 1, select Convection Bake, set temperature to 340ºF (171ºC), and set time to 16 minutes.
3. After 9 minutes, remove from the oven and add the shrimp, baby peas, and diced tomato to the baking pan. Mix well. Return the pan to the oven and continue cooking for 7 minutes more, or until the shrimp are done and the paella is bubbling.
4. When cooking is complete, remove from the oven. Cool for 5 minutes before serving.

250.Salmon & Caper Cakes

Servings: 2
Cooking Time: 15 Minutes + Chilling Time
Ingredients:

- 8 oz salmon, cooked
- 1 ½ oz potatoes, mashed
- A handful of capers
- 1 tbsp fresh parsley, chopped
- Zest of 1 lemon
- 1 ¾ oz plain flour

Directions:
1. Carefully flake the salmon. In a bowl, mix the salmon, zest, capers, dill, and mashed potatoes. Form small cakes from the mixture and dust them with flour; refrigerate for 60 minutes. Preheat Breville to 350 F. Press Start and cook the cakes for 10 minutes on AirFry function. Serve chilled.

251.Tasty Tuna Loaf

Servings: 6
Cooking Time: 40 Minutes
Ingredients:
- Nonstick cooking spray
- 12 oz. can chunk white tuna in water, drain & flake
- ¾ cup bread crumbs
- 1 onion, chopped fine
- 2 eggs, beaten
- ¼ cup milk
- ½ tsp fresh lemon juice
- ½ tsp dill
- 1 tbsp. fresh parsley, chopped
- ½ tsp salt
- ½ tsp pepper

Directions:
1. Place rack in position 1 of the oven. Spray a 9-inch loaf pan with cooking spray.
2. In a large bowl, combine all ingredients until thoroughly mixed. Spread evenly in prepared pan.
3. Set oven to bake on 350°F for 45 minutes. After 5 minutes, place the pan in the oven and cook 40 minutes, or until top is golden brown. Slice and serve.

Nutrition Info: Calories 169, Total Fat 5g, Saturated Fat 1g, Total Carbs 13g, Net Carbs 12g, Protein 18g, Sugar 3g, Fiber 1g, Sodium 540mg, Potassium 247mg, Phosphorus 202mg

252.Fish Tacos

Servings: 6
Cooking Time: 10 To 15 Minutes
Ingredients:
- 1 tablespoon avocado oil
- 1 tablespoon Cajun seasoning
- 4 (5 to 6 ounce / 142 to 170 g) tilapia fillets
- 1 (14-ounce / 397-g) package coleslaw mix
- 12 corn tortillas
- 2 limes, cut into wedges

Directions:
1. Line the baking pan with parchment paper.
2. In a shallow bowl, stir together the avocado oil and Cajun seasoning to make a marinade. Place the tilapia fillets into the bowl, turning to coat evenly.
3. Put the fillets in the baking pan in a single layer.
4. Put the air fryer basket on the baking pan and slide into Rack Position 2, select Air Fry, set temperature to 375ºF (190ºC), and set time to 10 minutes.
5. When cooked, the fish should be flaky. If necessary, continue cooking for 5 minutes more. Remove the fish from the oven to a plate.
6. Assemble the tacos: Spoon some of the coleslaw mix into each tortilla and top each with $^1/_3$ of a tilapia fillet. Squeeze some lime juice over the top of each taco and serve immediately.

253. Salmon Fritters

Ingredients:
- 2 tbsp. garam masala
- 1 lb. fileted Salmon
- 3 tsp ginger finely chopped
- 1-2 tbsp. fresh coriander leaves
- 2 or 3 green chilies finely chopped
- 1 ½ tbsp. lemon juice
- Salt and pepper to taste

Directions:
1. Mix the ingredients in a clean bowl.
2. Mold this mixture into round and flat French Cuisine Galettes.
3. Wet the French Cuisine Galettes slightly with water.
4. Pre heat the oven at 160 degrees Fahrenheit for 5 minutes. Place the French Cuisine Galettes in the fry basket and let them cook for another 25 minutes at the same temperature. Keep rolling them over to get a uniform cook. Serve either with mint sauce or ketchup.

254. Cheesy Tuna Patties

Servings: 4
Cooking Time: 17 To 18 Minutes
Ingredients:
- Tuna Patties:
- 1 pound (454 g) canned tuna, drained
- 1 egg, whisked
- 2 tablespoons shallots, minced
- 1 garlic clove, minced
- 1 cup grated Romano cheese
- Sea salt and ground black pepper, to taste
- 1 tablespoon sesame oil
- Cheese Sauce:

- 1 tablespoon butter
- 1 cup beer
- 2 tablespoons grated Colby cheese

Directions:
1. Mix together the canned tuna, whisked egg, shallots, garlic, cheese, salt, and pepper in a large bowl and stir to incorporate.
2. Divide the tuna mixture into four equal portions and form each portion into a patty with your hands. Refrigerate the patties for 2 hours.
3. When ready, brush both sides of each patty with sesame oil, then place in the baking pan.
4. Slide the baking pan into Rack Position 1, select Convection Bake, set temperature to 360ºF (182ºC), and set time to 14 minutes.
5. Flip the patties halfway through the cooking time.
6. Meanwhile, melt the butter in a saucepan over medium heat.
7. Pour in the beer and whisk constantly, or until it begins to bubble. Add the grated Colby cheese and mix well. Continue cooking for 3 to 4 minutes, or until the cheese melts. Remove from the heat.
8. When cooking is complete, the patties should be lightly browned and cooked through. Remove the patties from the oven to a plate. Drizzle them with the cheese sauce and serve immediately.

255. Flavorful Baked Halibut

Servings: 4
Cooking Time: 12 Minutes
Ingredients:
- 1 lb halibut fillets
- 1/4 tsp garlic powder
- 1/4 tsp paprika
- 1/4 tsp smoked paprika
- 1/4 tsp pepper
- 1/4 cup olive oil
- 1 lemon juice
- 1/2 tsp salt

Directions:
1. Fit the oven with the rack in position
2. Place fish fillets into the baking dish.
3. In a small bowl, mix lemon juice, oil, paprika, smoked paprika, garlic powder, and salt.
4. Brush lemon juice mixture over fish fillets.
5. Set to bake at 425 F for 17 minutes. After 5 minutes place the baking dish in the preheated oven.
6. Serve and enjoy.
Nutrition Info: Calories 236 Fat 15.3 g Carbohydrates 0.4 g Sugar 0.1 g Protein 24 g Cholesterol 36 mg

256.Crispy Paprika Fish Fillets(2)

Servings: 4
Cooking Time: 15 Minutes
Ingredients:
- 1/2 cup seasoned breadcrumbs
- 1 tablespoon balsamic vinegar
- 1/2 teaspoon seasoned salt
- 1 teaspoon paprika
- 1/2 teaspoon ground black pepper
- 1 teaspoon celery seed
- 2 fish fillets, halved
- 1 egg, beaten

Directions:
1.   Preparing the Ingredients. Add the breadcrumbs, vinegar, salt, paprika, ground black pepper, and celery seeds to your food processor. Process for about 30 seconds.
2.   Coat the fish fillets with the beaten egg; then, coat them with the breadcrumbs mixture.
3.   Air Frying. Cook at 350 degrees F for about 15 minutes.

257.Crispy Crab And Fish Cakes

Servings: 4
Cooking Time: 12 Minutes
Ingredients:
- 8 ounces (227 g) imitation crab meat
- 4 ounces (113 g) leftover cooked fish (such as cod, pollock, or haddock)
- 2 tablespoons minced celery
- 2 tablespoons minced green onion
- 2 tablespoons light mayonnaise
- 1 tablespoon plus 2 teaspoons Worcestershire sauce
- ¾ cup crushed saltine cracker crumbs
- 2 teaspoons dried parsley flakes
- 1 teaspoon prepared yellow mustard
- ½ teaspoon garlic powder
- ½ teaspoon dried dill weed, crushed
- ½ teaspoon Old Bay seasoning
- ½ cup panko bread crumbs
- Cooking spray

Directions:
1.   Pulse the crab meat and fish in a food processor until finely chopped.
2.   Transfer the meat mixture to a large bowl, along with the celery, green onion, mayo, Worcestershire sauce, cracker crumbs, parsley flakes, mustard, garlic powder, dill weed, and Old Bay seasoning. Stir to mix well.
3.   Scoop out the meat mixture and form into 8 equal-sized patties with your hands.
4.   Place the panko bread crumbs on a plate. Roll the patties in the bread crumbs until they are evenly coated on both sides. Put the patties in the baking pan and spritz them with cooking spray.
5.   Slide the baking pan into Rack Position 1, select Convection Bake, set temperature to 390ºF (199ºC), and set time to 12 minutes.
6.   Flip the patties halfway through the cooking time.
7.   When cooking is complete, they should be golden brown and cooked through. Remove the pan from the oven. Divide the patties among four plates and serve.

258.Lobster Tails With Lemon-garlic Sauce

Servings: 4
Cooking Time: 15 Minutes
Ingredients:
- 1 lb lobster tails
- 1 garlic clove, minced
- 1 tbsp butter
- Salt and black pepper to taste
- ½ tbsp lemon Juice

Directions:
1.   Add all the ingredients to a food processor, except for lobster and blend well. Wash lobster and halve using meat knife; clean the skin of the lobster and cover with the marinade.
2.   Preheat your Breville to 380 F. Place the lobster in the cooking basket and press Start. Cook for 10 minutes on AirFry function. Serve with fresh herbs.

259.Blackened Mahi Mahi

Servings: 4
Cooking Time: 12 Minutes
Ingredients:
- 4 mahi-mahi fillets
- 1 tsp cumin
- 1 tsp paprika
- 1/2 tsp cayenne pepper
- 1 tsp oregano
- 1 tsp garlic powder
- 1 tsp onion powder
- 1/2 tsp pepper
- 3 tbsp olive oil
- 1/2 tsp salt

Directions:
1.   Fit the oven with the rack in position
2.   Brush fish fillets with oil and place them into the baking dish.
3.   Mix together the remaining ingredients and sprinkle over fish fillets.
4.   Set to bake at 450 F for 17 minutes. After 5 minutes place the baking dish in the preheated oven.

5. Serve and enjoy.
Nutrition Info: Calories 189 Fat 11.7 g
Carbohydrates 2.1 g Sugar 0.5 g Protein 19.4 g
Cholesterol 86 mg

260.Tilapia Meunière With Vegetables

Servings: 4
Cooking Time: 20 Minutes
Ingredients:
- 10 ounces (283 g) Yukon Gold potatoes, sliced ¼-inch thick
- 5 tablespoons unsalted butter, melted, divided
- 1 teaspoon kosher salt, divided
- 4 (8-ounce / 227-g) tilapia fillets
- ½ pound (227 g) green beans, trimmed
- Juice of 1 lemon
- 2 tablespoons chopped fresh parsley, for garnish

Directions:
1. In a large bowl, drizzle the potatoes with 2 tablespoons of melted butter and ¼ teaspoon of kosher salt. Transfer the potatoes to the baking pan.
2. Slide the baking pan into Rack Position 2, select Roast, set temperature to 375ºF (190ºC), and set time to 20 minutes.
3. Meanwhile, season both sides of the fillets with ½ teaspoon of kosher salt. Put the green beans in the medium bowl and sprinkle with the remaining ¼ teaspoon of kosher salt and 1 tablespoon of butter, tossing to coat.
4. After 10 minutes, remove from the oven and push the potatoes to one side. Put the fillets in the middle of the pan and add the green beans on the other side. Drizzle the remaining 2 tablespoons of butter over the fillets. Return the pan to the oven and continue cooking, or until the fish flakes easily with a fork and the green beans are crisp-tender.
5. When cooked, remove from the oven. Drizzle the lemon juice over the fillets and sprinkle the parsley on top for garnish. Serve hot.

261.Air-fried Scallops

Servings: 2
Cooking Time: 12 Minutes
Ingredients:
- $^1/_3$ cup shallots, chopped
- 1½ tablespoons olive oil
- 1½ tablespoons coconut aminos
- 1 tablespoon Mediterranean seasoning mix
- ½ tablespoon balsamic vinegar
- ½ teaspoon ginger, grated
- 1 clove garlic, chopped
- 1 pound (454 g) scallops, cleanedCooking spray
- Belgian endive, for garnish

Directions:
1. Place all the ingredients except the scallops and Belgian endive in a small skillet over medium heat and stir to combine. Let this mixture simmer for about 2 minutes.
2. Remove the mixture from the skillet to a large bowl and set aside to cool.
3. Add the scallops, coating them all over, then transfer to the refrigerator to marinate for at least 2 hours.
4. When ready, place the scallops in the air fryer basket in a single layer and spray with cooking spray.
5. Put the air fryer basket on the baking pan and slide into Rack Position 2, select Air Fry, set temperature to 345ºF (174ºC), and set time to 10 minutes.
6. Flip the scallops halfway through the cooking time.
7. When cooking is complete, the scallops should be tender and opaque. Remove from the oven and serve garnished with the Belgian endive.

262.Simple Lemon Salmon

Servings: 2
Cooking Time: 20 Minutes
Ingredients:
- 2 salmon fillets
- Salt to taste
- Zest of a lemon

Directions:
1. Spray the fillets with olive oil and rub them with salt and lemon zest. Line baking paper in a baking dish. Cook the fillets in your for 10 minutes at 360 F on Air Fry, turning once.

263.Italian Cod

Servings: 4
Cooking Time: 20 Minutes
Ingredients:
- 1 1/2 lbs cod fillet
- 1/4 cup olives, sliced
- 1 lb cherry tomatoes, halved
- 2 garlic cloves, crushed
- 1 small onion, chopped
- 1 tbsp olive oil
- 1/4 cup of water
- 1 tsp Italian seasoning
- Pepper
- Salt

Directions:
1. Fit the oven with the rack in position
2. Place fish fillets, olives, tomatoes, garlic, and onion in a baking dish. Drizzle with oil.

3. Sprinkle with Italian seasoning, pepper, and salt. Pour water into the dish.
4. Set to bake at 400 F for 25 minutes. After 5 minutes place the baking dish in the preheated oven.
5. Serve and enjoy.
Nutrition Info: Calories 210 Fat 6.5 g Carbohydrates 7.2 g Sugar 3.8 g Protein 31.7 g Cholesterol 84 mg

264.Mediterranean Sole

Servings: 6
Cooking Time: 20 Minutes
Ingredients:
- Nonstick cooking spray
- 2 tbsp. olive oil
- 8 scallions, sliced thin
- 2 cloves garlic, diced fine
- 4 tomatoes, chopped
- ½ cup dry white wine
- 2 tbsp. fresh parsley, chopped fine
- 1 tsp oregano
- 1 tsp pepper
- 2 lbs. sole, cut in 6 pieces
- 4 oz. feta cheese, crumbled

Directions:
1. Place the rack in position 1 of the oven. Spray an 8x11-inch baking dish with cooking spray.
2. Heat the oil in a medium skillet over medium heat. Add scallions and garlic and cook until tender, stirring frequently.
3. Add the tomatoes, wine, parsley, oregano, and pepper. Stir to mix. Simmer for 5 minutes, or until sauce thickens. Remove from heat.
4. Pour half the sauce on the bottom of the prepared dish. Lay fish on top then pour remaining sauce over the top. Sprinkle with feta.
5. Set the oven to bake on 400°F for 25 minutes. After 5 minutes, place the baking dish on the rack and cook 15-18 minutes or until fish flakes easily with a fork. Serve immediately.
Nutrition Info: Calories 220, Total Fat 12g, Saturated Fat 4g, Total Carbs 6g, Net Carbs 4g, Protein 22g, Sugar 4g, Fiber 2g, Sodium 631mg, Potassium 540mg, Phosphorus 478mg

265.Lemon-garlic Butter Lobster

Servings: 2
Cooking Time: 15 Minutes
Ingredients:
- 4 oz lobster tails
- 1 tsp garlic, minced
- 1 tbsp butter
- Salt and black pepper to taste
- ½ tbsp lemon Juice

Directions:
1. Add all the ingredients to a food processor except for lobster and blend well. Wash lobster and halve using a meat knife; clean the skin of the lobster and cover with the marinade.
2. Preheat your to 380 F on Air Fry function. Place the lobster in the cooking basket and fit in the baking tray; cook for 10 minutes. Serve with fresh herbs.

266.Oyster Club Sandwich

Ingredients:
- 2 slices of white bread
- 1 tbsp. softened butter
- ½ lb. shelled oyster
- 1 small capsicum
- For Barbeque Sauce:
- ¼ tbsp. Worcestershire sauce
- ½ tsp. olive oil
- ½ flake garlic crushed
- ¼ cup chopped onion
- ¼ tsp. mustard powder
- 1 tbsp. tomato ketchup
- ½ tbsp. sugar
- ¼ tbsp. red chili sauce
- ½ cup water.
- A pinch of salt and black pepper to taste

Directions:
1. Take the slices of bread and remove the edges. Now cut the slices horizontally. Cook the ingredients for the sauce and wait till it thickens. Now, add the oyster to the sauce and stir till it obtains the flavors.
2. Roast the capsicum and peel the skin off. Cut the capsicum into slices. Mix the ingredients together and apply it to the bread slices. Pre-heat the oven for 5 minutes at 300 Fahrenheit. Open the basket of the Fryer and place the prepared Classic Sandwiches in it such that no two Classic Sandwiches are touching each other. Now keep the fryer at 250 degrees for around 15 minutes.
3. Turn the Classic Sandwiches in between the cooking process to cook both slices. Serve the Classic Sandwiches with tomato ketchup or mint sauce.

267.Tropical Shrimp Skewers

Servings: 4
Cooking Time: 5 Minutes
Ingredients:
- 1 tbsp. lime juice
- 1 tbsp. honey
- ¼ tsp red pepper flakes
- ¼ tsp pepper
- ¼ tsp ginger
- Nonstick cooking spray

- 1 lb. medium shrimp, peel, devein & leave tails on
- 2 cups peaches, drain & chop
- ½ green bell pepper, chopped fine
- ¼ cup scallions, chopped

Directions:
1. Soak 8 small wooden skewers in water for 15 minutes.
2. In a small bowl, whisk together lime juice, honey and spices. Transfer 2 tablespoons of the mixture to a medium bowl.
3. Place the baking pan in position 2 of the oven. Lightly spray fryer basket with cooking spray. Set oven to broil on 400°F for 10 minutes.
4. Thread 5 shrimp on each skewer and brush both sides with marinade. Place in basket and after 5 minutes, place on the baking pan. Cook 4-5 minutes or until shrimp turn pink.
5. Add peaches, bell pepper, and scallions to reserved honey mixture, mix well. Divide salsa evenly between serving plates and top with 2 skewers each. Serve immediately.

Nutrition Info: Calories 181, Total Fat 1g, Saturated Fat 0g, Total Carbs 27g, Net Carbs 25g, Protein 16g, Sugar 21g, Fiber 2g, Sodium 650mg, Potassium 288mg, Phosphorus 297mg

268.Crab Cakes With Bell Peppers

Servings: 4
Cooking Time: 10 Minutes
Ingredients:
- 8 ounces (227 g) jumbo lump crab meat
- 1 egg, beaten
- Juice of ½ lemon
- $^1/_3$ cup bread crumbs
- ¼ cup diced green bell pepper
- ¼ cup diced red bell pepper
- ¼ cup mayonnaise
- 1 tablespoon Old Bay seasoning
- 1 teaspoon flour
- Cooking spray

Directions:
1. Make the crab cakes: Place all the ingredients except the flour and oil in a large bowl and stir until well incorporated.
2. Divide the crab mixture into four equal portions and shape each portion into a patty with your hands. Top each patty with a sprinkle of ¼ teaspoon of flour.
3. Arrange the crab cakes in the air fryer basket and spritz them with cooking spray.
4. Put the air fryer basket on the baking pan and slide into Rack Position 2, select Air Fry, set temperature to 375ºF (190ºC), and set time to 10 minutes.
5. Flip the crab cakes halfway through.

6. When cooking is complete, the cakes should be cooked through. Remove from the oven and divide the crab cakes among four plates and serve.

269.Spicy Grilled Halibut

Servings: 4
Cooking Time: 10 Minutes
Ingredients:
- ½ cup fresh lemon juice
- 2 jalapeno peppers, seeded & chopped fine
- 4 6 oz. halibut fillets
- Nonstick cooking spray
- ¼ cup cilantro, chopped

Directions:
1. In a small bowl, combine lemon juice and chilies, mix well.
2. Place fish in a large Ziploc bag and add marinade. Toss to coat. Refrigerate 30 minutes.
3. Lightly spray the baking pan with cooking spray. Set oven to broil on 400°F for 15 minutes.
4. After 5 minutes, lay fish on the pan and place in position 2 of the oven. Cook 10 minutes, or until fish flakes easily with a fork. Turn fish over and brush with marinade halfway through cooking time.
5. Sprinkle with cilantro before serving.

Nutrition Info: Calories 328, Total Fat 24g, Saturated Fat 4g, Total Carbs 3g, Net Carbs 3g, Protein 25g, Sugar 1g, Fiber 0g, Sodium 137mg, Potassium 510mg, Phosphorus 284mg

270.Sesame Seeds Coated Fish

Servings: 5
Cooking Time: 8 Minutes
Ingredients:
- 3 tablespoons plain flour
- 2 eggs
- ½ cup sesame seeds, toasted
- ½ cup breadcrumbs
- 1/8 teaspoon dried rosemary, crushed
- Pinch of salt
- Pinch of black pepper
- 3 tablespoons olive oil
- 5 frozen fish fillets (white fish of your choice)

Directions:
1. Preparing the Ingredients. In a shallow dish, place flour. In a second shallow dish, beat the eggs. In a third shallow dish, add remaining ingredients except fish fillets and mix till a crumbly mixture forms.
2. Coat the fillets with flour and shake off the excess flour.
3. Next, dip the fillets in the egg.

4. Then coat the fillets with sesame seeds mixture generously.
5. Preheat the air fryer oven to 390 degrees F.
6. Air Frying. Line an Air fryer rack/basket with a piece of foil. Arrange the fillets into prepared basket.
7. Cook for about 14 minutes, flipping once after 10 minutes.

271.Baked Garlic Paprika Halibut

Servings: 4
Cooking Time: 12 Minutes
Ingredients:
- 1 lb halibut fillets
- 1/2 tsp smoked paprika
- 1/4 cup olive oil
- 1/4 tsp garlic powder
- Pepper
- Salt
Directions:
1. Fit the oven with the rack in position
2. Place fish fillets in a baking dish.
3. In a small bowl, mix together oil, garlic powder, paprika, pepper, and salt.
4. Brush fish fillets with oil mixture.
5. Set to bake at 425 F for 17 minutes. After 5 minutes place the baking dish in the preheated oven.
6. Serve and enjoy.
Nutrition Info: Calories 235 Fat 15.3 g Carbohydrates 0.3 g Sugar 0.1 g Protein 23.9 g Cholesterol 36 mg

272.Lemon Butter Shrimp

Servings: 4
Cooking Time: 12 Minutes
Ingredients:
- 1 1/4 lbs shrimp, peeled & deveined
- 2 tbsp fresh parsley, chopped
- 2 tbsp fresh lemon juice
- 1 tbsp garlic, minced
- 1/4 cup butter
- Pepper
- Salt
Directions:
1. Fit the oven with the rack in position
2. Add shrimp into the baking dish.
3. Melt butter in a pan over low heat. Add garlic and sauté for 30 seconds. Stir in lemon juice.
4. Pour melted butter mixture over shrimp. Season with pepper and salt.
5. Set to bake at 350 F for 17 minutes. After 5 minutes place the baking dish in the preheated oven.
6. Garnish with parsley and serve.

Nutrition Info: Calories 276 Fat 14 g Carbohydrates 3.2 g Sugar 0.2 g Protein 32.7 g Cholesterol 329 mg

273.Baked Flounder Fillets

Servings: 2
Cooking Time: 12 Minutes
Ingredients:
- 2 flounder fillets, patted dry
- 1 egg
- ½ teaspoon Worcestershire sauce
- ¼ cup almond flour
- ¼ cup coconut flour
- ½ teaspoon coarse sea salt
- ½ teaspoon lemon pepper
- ¼ teaspoon chili powder
- Cooking spray
Directions:
1. In a shallow bowl, beat together the egg with Worcestershire sauce until well incorporated.
2. In another bowl, thoroughly combine the almond flour, coconut flour, sea salt, lemon pepper, and chili powder.
3. Dredge the fillets in the egg mixture, shaking off any excess, then roll in the flour mixture to coat well.
4. Spritz the baking pan with cooking spray. Place the fillets in the pan.
5. Slide the baking pan into Rack Position 1, select Convection Bake, set temperature to 390ºF (199ºC), and set time to 12 minutes.
6. After 7 minutes, remove from the oven and flip the fillets and spray with cooking spray. Return the pan to the oven and continue cooking for 5 minutes, or until the fish is flaky.
7. When cooking is complete, remove from the oven and serve warm.

274.Prawn French Cuisine Galette

Ingredients:
- 2 tbsp. garam masala
- 1 lb. minced prawn
- 3 tsp ginger finely chopped
- 1-2 tbsp. fresh coriander leaves
- 2 or 3 green chilies finely chopped
- 1 ½ tbsp. lemon juice
- Salt and pepper to taste
Directions:
1. Mix the ingredients in a clean bowl.
2. Mold this mixture into round and flat French Cuisine Galettes.
3. Wet the French Cuisine Galettes slightly with water.
4. Pre heat the oven at 160 degrees Fahrenheit for 5 minutes. Place the French Cuisine Galettes in the

fry basket and let them cook for another 25 minutes at the same temperature. Keep rolling them over to get a uniform cook. Serve either with mint sauce or ketchup.

275.Thyme Rosemary Shrimp

Servings: 4
Cooking Time: 10 Minutes
Ingredients:
- 1 lb shrimp, peeled and deveined
- 1/2 tbsp fresh rosemary, chopped
- 1 tbsp olive oil
- 2 garlic cloves, minced
- 1/2 tbsp fresh thyme, chopped
- Pepper
- Salt

Directions:
1. Fit the oven with the rack in position
2. Add shrimp and remaining ingredients in a large bowl and toss well.
3. Pour shrimp mixture into the baking dish.
4. Set to bake at 400 F for 15 minutes. After 5 minutes place the baking dish in the preheated oven.
5. Serve and enjoy.
Nutrition Info: Calories 169 Fat 5.5 g Carbohydrates 2.7 g Sugar 0 g Protein 26 g Cholesterol 239 mg

276.Parmesan-crusted Salmon Patties

Servings: 4
Cooking Time: 13 Minutes
Ingredients:
- 1 pound (454 g) salmon, chopped into ½-inch pieces
- 2 tablespoons coconut flour
- 2 tablespoons grated Parmesan cheese
- 1½ tablespoons milk
- ½ white onion, peeled and finely chopped
- ½ teaspoon butter, at room temperature
- ½ teaspoon chipotle powder
- ½ teaspoon dried parsley flakes
- $^1/_3$ teaspoon ground black pepper
- $^1/_3$ teaspoon smoked cayenne pepper
- 1 teaspoon fine sea salt

Directions:
1. Put all the ingredients for the salmon patties in a bowl and stir to combine well.
2. Scoop out 2 tablespoons of the salmon mixture and shape into a patty with your palm, about ½ inch thick. Repeat until all the mixture is used. Transfer to the refrigerator for about 2 hours until firm.
3. When ready, arrange the salmon patties in the baking pan.

4. Slide the baking pan into Rack Position 1, select Convection Bake, set temperature to 395ºF (202ºC), and set time to 13 minutes.
5. Flip the patties halfway through the cooking time.
6. When cooking is complete, the patties should be golden brown. Remove from the oven and cool for 5 minutes before serving.

277.Salmon Fries

Ingredients:
- 1 lb. boneless salmon filets
- 2 cup dry breadcrumbs
- 2 tsp. oregano
- 2 tsp. red chili flakes
- 1 ½ tbsp. ginger-garlic paste
- 4 tbsp. lemon juice
- 2 tsp. salt
- 1 tsp. pepper powder
- 1 tsp. red chili powder
- 6 tbsp. corn flour
- 4 eggs

Directions:
1. Mix all the ingredients for the marinade and put the salmon filets inside and let it rest overnight. Mix the breadcrumbs, oregano and red chili flakes well and place the marinated Oregano Fingers on this mixture. Cover it with plastic wrap and leave it till right before you serve to cook.
2. Pre heat the oven at 160 degrees Fahrenheit for 5 minutes.
3. Place the Oregano Fingers in the fry basket and close it. Let them cook at the same temperature for another 15 minutes or so. Toss the Oregano Fingers well so that they are cooked uniformly.

278.Spinach Scallops

Servings: 2
Cooking Time: 10 Minutes
Ingredients:
- 8 sea scallops
- 1 tbsp fresh basil, chopped
- 1 tbsp tomato paste
- 3/4 cup heavy cream
- 12 oz frozen spinach, thawed and drained
- 1 tsp garlic, minced
- 1/2 tsp pepper
- 1/2 tsp salt

Directions:
1. Fit the oven with the rack in position
2. Layer spinach in the baking dish.
3. Spray scallops with cooking spray and season with pepper and salt.

4. Place scallops on top of spinach.
5. In a small bowl, mix garlic, basil, tomato paste, whipping cream, pepper, and salt and pour over scallops and spinach.
6. Set to bake at 350 F for 15 minutes. After 5 minutes place the baking dish in the preheated oven.
7. Serve and enjoy.
Nutrition Info: Calories 310 Fat 18.3 g Carbohydrates 12.6 g Sugar 1.7 g Protein 26.5 g Cholesterol 101 mg

279.Piri-piri King Prawns

Servings: 2
Cooking Time: 8 Minutes
Ingredients:
- 12 king prawns, rinsed
- 1 tablespoon coconut oil
- Salt and ground black pepper, to taste
- 1 teaspoon onion powder
- 1 teaspoon garlic paste
- 1 teaspoon curry powder
- ½ teaspoon piri piri powder
- ½ teaspoon cumin powder

Directions:
1. Combine all the ingredients in a large bowl and toss until the prawns are completely coated. Place the prawns in the air fryer basket.
2. Put the air fryer basket on the baking pan and slide into Rack Position 2, select Air Fry, set temperature to 360ºF (182ºC), and set time to 8 minutes.
3. Flip the prawns halfway through the cooking time.
4. When cooking is complete, the prawns will turn pink. Remove from the oven and serve hot.

280.Homemade Fish Sticks

Servings: 8 Fish Sticks
Cooking Time: 8 Minutes
Ingredients:
- 8 ounces (227 g) fish fillets (pollock or cod), cut into ½×3-inch strips
- Salt, to taste (optional)
- ½ cup plain bread crumbs
- Cooking spray

Directions:
1. Season the fish strips with salt to taste, if desired.
2. Place the bread crumbs on a plate. Roll the fish strips in the bread crumbs to coat. Spritz the fish strips with cooking spray.
3. Arrange the fish strips in the air fryer basket in a single layer.

4. Put the air fryer basket on the baking pan and slide into Rack Position 2, select Air Fry, set temperature to 390ºF (199ºC), and set time to 8 minutes.
5. When cooking is complete, they should be golden brown. Remove from the oven and cool for 5 minutes before serving.

281.Rosemary Garlic Shrimp

Servings: 4
Cooking Time: 10 Minutes
Ingredients:
- 1 lb shrimp, peeled and deveined
- 2 garlic cloves, minced
- 1/2 tbsp fresh rosemary, chopped
- 1 tbsp olive oil
- Pepper
- Salt

Directions:
1. Fit the oven with the rack in position
2. Add shrimp and remaining ingredients in a large bowl and toss well.
3. Pour shrimp mixture into the baking dish.
4. Set to bake at 400 F for 15 minutes. After 5 minutes place the baking dish in the preheated oven.
5. Serve and enjoy.
Nutrition Info: Calories 168 Fat 5.5 g Carbohydrates 2.5 g Sugar 0 g Protein 26 g Cholesterol 239 mg

282.Easy Shrimp Fajitas

Servings: 10
Cooking Time: 20 Minutes
Ingredients:
- 1 lb shrimp
- 1 tbsp olive oil
- 2 bell peppers, diced
- 2 tbsp taco seasoning
- 1/2 cup onion, diced

Directions:
1. Fit the oven with the rack in position 2.
2. Add shrimp and remaining ingredients into the bowl and toss well.
3. Add shrimp mixture to the air fryer basket then place an air fryer basket in baking pan.
4. Place a baking pan on the oven rack. Set to air fry at 390 F for 20 minutes.
5. Serve and enjoy.
Nutrition Info: Calories 76 Fat 2.2 g Carbohydrates 3 g Sugar 1.4 g Protein 10.6 g Cholesterol 96 mg

283.Parmesan Tilapia Fillets

Servings: 4

Cooking Time: 15 Minutes

Ingredients:

- ¾ cup Parmesan cheese, grated
- 1 tbsp olive oil
- 1 tsp paprika
- 1 tbsp fresh parsley, chopped
- ¼ tsp garlic powder
- ¼ tsp salt
- 4 tilapia fillets

Directions:

1. Preheat Breville on AirFry function to 350 F. In a bowl, mix parsley, Parmesan cheese, garlic, salt, and paprika. Coat in the tilapia fillets and place them in a lined baking sheet. Drizzle with the olive oil press Start. Cook cook for 8-10 minutes until golden. Serve warm.

284.Crab Cakes

Servings: 4
Cooking Time: 10 Minutes

Ingredients:

- 8 ounces jumbo lump crabmeat
- 1 tablespoon Old Bay Seasoning
- ⅓ cup bread crumbs
- ¼ cup diced red bell pepper
- ¼ cup diced green bell pepper
- 1 egg
- ¼ cup mayonnaise
- Juice of ½ lemon
- 1 teaspoon flour
- Cooking oil

Directions:

1. Preparing the Ingredients. In a large bowl, combine the crabmeat, Old Bay Seasoning, bread crumbs, red bell pepper, green bell pepper, egg, mayo, and lemon juice. Mix gently to combine.
2. Form the mixture into 4 patties. Sprinkle ¼ teaspoon of flour on top of each patty.
3. Air Frying. Place the crab cakes in the air fryer oven. Spray them with cooking oil. Cook for 10 minutes.
4. Serve.

285.Garlic-butter Catfish

Servings: 2
Cooking Time: 20 Minutes

Ingredients:

- 2 catfish fillets
- 2 tsp blackening seasoning
- Juice of 1 lime
- 2 tbsp butter, melted
- 1 garlic clove, mashed
- 2 tbsp cilantro

Directions:

1. In a bowl, blend in garlic, lime juice, cilantro, and butter. Pour half of the mixture over the fillets and sprinkle with blackening seasoning. Place the fillets in the basket and fit in the baking tray; cook for 15 minutes at 360 F on Air Fry function. Serve the fish with remaining sauce.

APPETIZERS AND SIDE DISHES

286.Creamy Fennel(2)

Servings: 4
Cooking Time: 8 Minutes
Ingredients:
- 2 big fennel bulbs; sliced
- ½ cup coconut cream
- 2 tbsp. butter; melted
- Salt and black pepper to taste.

Directions:
1. In a pan that fits the air fryer, combine all the ingredients, toss, introduce in the machine and cook at 370°F for 12 minutes
2. Divide between plates and serve as a side dish.

Nutrition Info: Calories: 151; Fat: 3g; Fiber: 2g; Carbs: 4g; Protein: 6g

287.Lemon Garlic Brussels Sprouts

Servings: 2
Cooking Time: 12 Minutes
Ingredients:
- 1/2 lb Brussels sprouts, rinse and pat dry with a paper towel
- 1/2 tsp garlic powder
- 1 tbsp lemon juice
- 1/4 tsp black pepper
- 1 tbsp olive oil
- 1/2 tsp salt

Directions:
1. Fit the oven with the rack in position 2.
2. Cut the stem of Brussels sprouts and cut each Brussels sprouts in half.
3. Transfer Brussels sprouts in a bowl and toss with garlic powder, olive oil, pepper, and salt.
4. Transfer Brussels sprouts in air fryer basket then place air fryer basket in baking pan.
5. Place baking pan on the oven rack. Set to air fry at 360 F for 12 minutes.
6. Drizzle with lemon juice and serve.

Nutrition Info: Calories 114 Fat 7.5 g Carbohydrates 11.2 g Sugar 2.8 g Protein 4.1 g Cholesterol 0 mg

288.Cod Nuggets

Servings: 5
Cooking Time: 8 Minutes
Ingredients:
- 1 cup all-purpose flour
- 2 eggs
- ¾ cup breadcrumbs
- Pinch of salt
- 2 tablespoons olive oil
- 1 lb. cod, cut into 1x2½-inch strips

Directions:
1. In a shallow dish, place the flour.
2. Crack the eggs in a second dish and beat well.
3. In a third dish, mix together the breadcrumbs, salt, and oil.
4. Coat the nuggets with flour, then dip into beaten eggs and finally, coat with the breadcrumbs.
5. Press "Power Button" of Air Fry Oven and turn the dial to select the "Air Fry" mode.
6. Press the Time button and again turn the dial to set the cooking time to 8 minutes.
7. Now push the Temp button and rotate the dial to set the temperature at 390 degrees F.
8. Press "Start/Pause" button to start.
9. When the unit beeps to show that it is preheated, open the lid.
10. Arrange the nuggets in "Air Fry Basket" and insert in the oven.
11. Serve warm.

Nutrition Info: Calories 323 Total Fat 9.2 g Saturated Fat 1.7 g Cholesterol 115 mg Sodium 245 mg Total Carbs 30.9 g Fiber 1.4 g Sugar 1.2 g Protein 27.7 g

289.Baked Vegetables

Servings: 6
Cooking Time: 30 Minutes
Ingredients:
- 2 zucchini, sliced
- 2 tomatoes, quartered
- 6 fresh basil leaves, sliced
- 2 tsp Italian seasoning
- 2 tbsp olive oil
- 1 eggplant, sliced
- 1 onion, sliced
- 1 bell pepper, cut into strips
- Pepper
- Salt

Directions:
1. Fit the oven with the rack in position
2. Add all ingredients except basil leaves into the bowl and toss well.
3. Transfer vegetable mixture in parchment-lined baking pan.
4. Set to bake at 400 F for 35 minutes. After 5 minutes place the baking pan in the preheated oven.
5. Garnish with basil and serve.

Nutrition Info: Calories 96 Fat 5.5 g Carbohydrates 11.7 g Sugar 6.4 g Protein 2.3 g Cholesterol 1 mg

290.Easy Parsnip Fries

Servings: 3

Cooking Time: 15 Minutes
Ingredients:
- 4 parsnips, sliced
- ¼ cup flour
- ¼ cup olive oil
- ¼ cup water
- A pinch of salt

Directions:
1. Preheat on Air Fry function to 390 F. In a bowl, add the flour, olive oil, water, and parsnips; mix to coat. Line the fries in the greased Air Fryer basket and fit in the baking tray. Cook for 15 minutes. Serve with yogurt and garlic dip.

291.Apple & Cinnamon Chips

Servings: 2
Cooking Time: 25 Minutes
Ingredients:
- 1 tsp sugar
- 1 tsp salt
- 1 whole apple, sliced
- ½ tsp cinnamon
- Confectioners' sugar for serving

Directions:
1. Preheat your Breville oven to 400 F on Bake function. In a bowl, mix cinnamon, salt, and sugar. Add in the apple slices and toss to coat. Transfer to a greased baking tray. Press Start and set the time to 10 minutes. When ready, dust with sugar and serve chilled.

292.Homemade Prosciutto Wrapped Cheese Sticks

Servings: 6
Cooking Time: 50 Minutes
Ingredients:
- 1 lb cheddar cheese
- 12 slices of prosciutto
- 1 cup flour
- 2 eggs, beaten
- 4 tbsp olive oil
- 1 cup breadcrumbs

Directions:
1. Cut the cheese into 6 equal sticks. Wrap each piece with 2 prosciutto slices. Place them in the freezer just enough to set. Preheat on Air Fry function to 390 F. Dip the croquettes into flour first, then in eggs, and coat with breadcrumbs. Drizzle the basket with oil and fit in the baking tray. Cook for 10 minutes or until golden. Serve.

293.Mashed Turnips

Servings: 4
Cooking Time: 5 Minutes
Ingredients:
- ½ cup chicken stock
- 4 turnips, peeled and chopped
- ¼ cup sour cream
- Salt and ground black pepper, to taste
- 1 yellow onion, peeled and chopped

Directions:
1. In the Instant Pot, mix the turnips with the stock and onion. Stir, cover and cook in manual setting for 5 minutes.
2. Release the pressure naturally, drain the turnips and transfer to a bowl. Mix them using a food processor and add salt and pepper to taste and sour cream. Mix again and serve.

Nutrition Info: Calories: 70, Fat: 1, Fiber: 4.6, Carbohydrate: 11.2, Proteins: 1.6

294.Honey-roasted Carrots With Sesame Seeds

Servings: 4
Cooking Time: 10 Minutes
Ingredients:
- 2 bags baby carrots
- 2 tablespoons olive oil
- 2 tablespoons honey
- Salt and pepper to taste
- 1 tablespoon soy sauce
- 1 tablespoon chopped fresh parsley
- 2 teaspoons sesame seeds

Directions:
1. Start by preheating toaster oven to 450°F.
2. Line a pan with parchment paper and put in oven while it heats.
3. In a small bowl, mix together oil and 1 tablespoon honey.
4. Drizzle honey mixture over carrots.
5. Sprinkle with salt and pepper.
6. Roast carrots for 10 minutes.
7. Mix soy sauce and remaining honey together and toss with carrots.
8. Sprinkle parsley and sesame seeds over carrots and serve.

Nutrition Info: Calories: 142, Sodium: 314 mg, Dietary Fiber: 3.5 g, Total Fat: 7.9 g, Total Carbs: 18.7 g, Protein: 1.3 g.

295.Rosemary & Thyme Roasted Fingerling Potatoes

Servings: 4
Cooking Time: 25 Minutes

Ingredients:
- 1 small bag baby fingerling potatoes
- 3 tablespoons olive oil
- Salt and pepper to taste
- 2 teaspoons rosemary
- 2 teaspoons thyme

Directions:
1. Start by preheating the toaster oven to 400°F.
2. Toss potatoes in olive oil and place on a baking sheet.
3. Pierce each potato to prevent overexpansion.
4. Sprinkle salt, pepper, rosemary, and thyme over the potatoes.
5. Roast for 25 minutes.

Nutrition Info: Calories: 123, Sodium: 3 mg, Dietary Fiber: 1.2 g, Total Fat: 10.7 g, Total Carbs: 7.5 g, Protein: 0.9 g.

296.Cabbage And Radishes Mix

Servings: 4
Cooking Time: 20 Minutes
Ingredients:
- 6 cups green cabbage; shredded
- ½ cup celery leaves; chopped.
- ¼ cup green onions; chopped.
- 6 radishes; sliced
- 3 tbsp. olive oil
- 2 tbsp. balsamic vinegar
- ½ tsp. hot paprika
- 1 tsp. lemon juice

Directions:
1. In your air fryer's pan, combine all the ingredients and toss well.
2. Introduce the pan in the fryer and cook at 380°F for 15 minutes. Divide between plates and serve as a side dish

Nutrition Info: Calories: 130; Fat: 4g; Fiber: 3g; Carbs: 4g; Protein: 7g

297.Delicious Chicken Wings With Alfredo Sauce

Servings: 4
Cooking Time: 60 Minutes
Ingredients:
- 1 ½ pounds chicken wings
- Salt and black pepper to taste
- ½ cup Alfredo sauce

Directions:
1. Preheat on Air Fry function to 370 F. Season the wings with salt and pepper. Arrange them on the greased basket without touching. Fit in the baking tray and cook for 20 minutes until no longer pink in the center. Work in batches if needed. Increase the

heat to 390 F and cook for 5 minutes more. Remove to a large bowl and drizzle with the Alfredo sauce. Serve.

298.French Beans With Toasted Almonds

Servings: 4
Cooking Time: 25 Minutes
Ingredients:
- 1 ½ lb French beans, trimmed
- Salt and black pepper to taste
- ½ pound shallots, chopped
- 3 tbsp olive oil
- ½ cup almonds, toasted

Directions:
1. Preheat on Air Fry function to 400 F. Blanch the French beans in filled with water pot over medium heat until tender, about 5-6 minutes. Remove with slotted spoon toa bowl and mix in olive oil, shallots, salt, and pepper. Add the mixture to a baking dish and cook in your for 10 minutes, shaking once or twice. Serve sprinkled with almonds.

299.Chili Beef Sticks

Servings: 3
Cooking Time: 10 Minutes
Ingredients:
- 1 lb ground beef
- 3 tbsp sugar
- A pinch garlic powder
- A pinch chili powder
- Salt to taste
- 1 tsp liquid smoke

Directions:
1. Place the meat, sugar, garlic powder, chili powder, salt, and liquid smoke in a bowl. Mix well. Mold out 4 sticks with your hands, place them on a plate, and refrigerate for 2 hours.
2. Select Bake function, adjust the temperature to 360 F, and press Start. Cook for 15 minutes.

300.Potatoes Au Gratin

Servings: 6
Cooking Time: 17 Minutes
Ingredients:
- ½ cup yellow onion, chopped
- 2 tablespoons butter
- 1 cup chicken stock
- 6 potatoes, peeled and sliced
- ½ cup sour cream
- Salt and ground black pepper, to taste
- 1 cup Monterey jack cheese, shredded
- For the topping:

- 3 tablespoons melted butter
- 1 cup breadcrumbs

Directions:
1. Put the Instant Pot in Saute mode, add the butter and melt. Add the onion, mix and cook for 5 minutes. Add the stock, salt and pepper and put the steamer basket in the Instant Pot also.
2. Add the potatoes, cover the Instant Pot and cook for 5 minutes in the Manual setting. In a bowl, mix 3 tablespoons of butter with breadcrumbs and mix well. Relieve the pressure of the Instant Pot, remove the steam basket and transfer the potatoes to a pan.
3. Pour the cream and cheese into the instant pot and mix. Add the potatoes and mix gently.
4. Spread breadcrumbs, mix everywhere, place on a preheated grill and cook for 7 minutes. Let cool for a few minutes and serve.

Nutrition Info: Calories: 340, Fat: 22, Fiber: 2, Carbohydrate: 32, Proteins: 11

301.Crispy Cinnamon Apple Chips

Servings: 4
Cooking Time: 10 Minutes
Ingredients:
- 2 apples, cored and cut into thin slices
- 2 heaped teaspoons ground cinnamon
- Cooking spray

Directions:
1. Spritz the air fryer basket with cooking spray.
2. In a medium bowl, sprinkle the apple slices with the cinnamon. Toss until evenly coated. Spread the coated apple slices on the pan in a single layer.
3. Put the air fryer basket on the baking pan and slide into Rack Position 2, select Air Fry, set temperature to 350ºF (180ºC) and set time to 10 minutes.
4. After 5 minutes, remove from the oven. Stir the apple slices and return to the oven to continue cooking.
5. When cooking is complete, the slices should be until crispy. Remove from the oven and let rest for 5 minutes before serving.

302.Parmesan Asparagus Fries

Servings: 4
Cooking Time: 6 Minutes
Ingredients:
- 2 egg whites
- ¼ cup water
- ¼ cup plus 2 tablespoons grated Parmesan cheese, divided
- ¾ cup panko bread crumbs
- ¼ teaspoon salt

- 12 ounces (340 g) fresh asparagus spears, woody ends trimmed
- Cooking spray

Directions:
1. In a shallow dish, whisk together the egg whites and water until slightly foamy. In a separate shallow dish, thoroughly combine ¼ cup of Parmesan cheese, bread crumbs, and salt.
2. Dip the asparagus in the egg white, then roll in the cheese mixture to coat well.
3. Place the asparagus in the air fryer basket in a single layer, leaving space between each spear. Spritz the asparagus with cooking spray.
4. Put the air fryer basket on the baking pan and slide into Rack Position 2, select Air Fry, set temperature to 390ºF (199ºC), and set time to 6 minutes.
5. When cooking is complete, the asparagus should be golden brown and crisp. Remove from the oven. Sprinkle with the remaining 2 tablespoons of cheese and serve hot.

303.Feta Butterbeans With Crispy Bacon

Servings: 2
Cooking Time: 10 Minutes
Ingredients:
- 1 (14 oz) can butter beans
- 1 tbsp chives
- 3 ½ oz feta, crumbled
- Black pepper to taste
- 1 tsp olive oil
- 3 ½ oz bacon, sliced

Directions:
1. Preheat on Air Fry function to 340 F. Blend beans, olive oil, and pepper in a blender. Arrange bacon slices on your Air fryer basket. Sprinkle chives on top and fit in the baking pan. Cook for 12 minutes. Add feta cheese to the bean mixture and stir. Serve bacon with the dip.

304.Philly Egg Rolls

Servings: 6
Cooking Time: 25 Minutes
Ingredients:
- Nonstick cooking spray
- ½ lb. lean ground beef
- ¼ tsp garlic powder
- ¼ tsp onion powder
- ¼ tsp salt
- ¼ tsp pepper
- ¾ cup green bell pepper, chopped
- ¾ cup onion, chopped
- 2 slices provolone cheese, torn into pieces

- 3 tbsp. cream cheese
- 6 square egg roll wrappers

Directions:

1. Place baking pan in position 2. Lightly spray fryer basket with cooking spray.
2. Heat a large skillet over med-high heat. Add beef, garlic powder, onion powder, salt and pepper. Stir to combine.
3. Add in bell pepper and onion and cook, stirring occasionally, until beef is no longer pink and vegetables are tender, about 6-8 minutes.
4. Remove from heat and drain fat. Add provolone and cream cheese and stir until melted and combined. Transfer to a large bowl.
5. Lay egg roll wrappers, one at a time, on a dry work surface. Spoon about 1/3 cup mixture in a row just below the center of the wrapper. Moisten edges with water. Fold the sides in towards the middle and roll up around filling.
6. Place egg rolls, seam side down in fryer basket. Spray lightly with cooking spray. Place the basket in the oven and set to air fry on 400°F for 10 minutes. Cook until golden brown, turning over halfway through cooking time. Serve immediately.

Nutrition Info: Calories 238, Total Fat 10g, Saturated Fat 5g, Total Carbs 21g, Net Carbs 20g, Protein 16g, Sugar 1g, Fiber 1g, Sodium 412mg, Potassium 206mg, Phosphorus 160mg

305.Vegetable & Walnut Stuffed Ham Rolls

Servings: 4
Cooking Time: 15 Minutes
Ingredients:

- 1 carrot, chopped
- 4 large ham slices
- ¼ cup walnuts, finely chopped
- 1 zucchini, chopped
- 1 garlic clove, minced
- 2 tbsp olive oil
- 1 tbsp ginger powder
- 2 tbsp fresh basil leaves, chopped
- Salt and black pepper to taste

Directions:

1. Heat olive oil in a pan over medium heat and sauté zucchini, carrot, garlic, and ginger for 5-6 minutes until tender. Stir in basil, walnuts, and salt.
2. Divide the mixture between ham slices and then fold one side above the filling and roll in. Transfer to a baking tray. Select Bake function, adjust the temperature to 360 F, and press Start. Bake the rolls for 8 minutes.

306.Winter Vegetables With Herbs

Servings: 2
Cooking Time: 20 Minutes
Ingredients:

- 1/2-pound broccoli florets
- 1 celery root, peeled and cut into 1-inch pieces
- 1 onion, cut into wedges
- 2 tablespoons unsalted butter, melted
- 1/2 cup chicken broth
- 1/4 cup tomato sauce
- 1 teaspoon parsley
- 1 teaspoon rosemary
- 1 teaspoon thyme

Directions:

1. Start by preheating your Air Fryer to 380 degrees F. Place all ingredients in a lightly greased casserole dish. Stir to combine well.
2. Bake in the preheated Air Fryer for 10 minutes. Gently stir the vegetables with a large spoon and cook for 5 minutes more.
3. Serve in individual bowls with a few drizzles of lemon juice.

Nutrition Info: 141 Calories; 13g Fat; 1g Carbs; 5g Protein; 9g Sugars; 6g Fiber

307.Spicy Tortilla Chips

Servings: 4
Cooking Time: 5 Minutes
Ingredients:

- ½ teaspoon ground cumin
- ½ teaspoon paprika
- ½ teaspoon chili powder
- ½ teaspoon salt
- Pinch cayenne pepper
- 8 (6-inch) corn tortillas, each cut into 6 wedges
- Cooking spray

Directions:

1. Lightly spritz the air fryer basket with cooking spray.
2. Stir together the cumin, paprika, chili powder, salt, and pepper in a small bowl.
3. Place the tortilla wedges in the basket in a single layer. Lightly mist them with cooking spray. Sprinkle the seasoning mixture on top of the tortilla wedges.
4. Put the air fryer basket on the baking pan and slide into Rack Position 2, select Air Fry, set temperature to 375ºF (190ºC), and set time to 5 minutes.
5. Stir the tortilla wedges halfway through the cooking time.
6. When cooking is complete, the chips should be lightly browned and crunchy. Remove from the oven. Let the tortilla chips cool for 5 minutes and serve.

308.Broiled Prosciutto-wrapped Pears

Servings: 8
Cooking Time: 6 Minutes
Ingredients:
- 2 large, ripe Anjou pears
- 4 thin slices Parma prosciutto
- 2 teaspoons aged balsamic vinegar

Directions:
1. Peel the pears. Slice into 8 wedges and cut out the core from each wedge.
2. Cut the prosciutto into 8 long strips. Wrap each pear wedge with a strip of prosciutto. Place the wrapped pears in the air fryer basket.
3. Put the air fryer basket on the baking pan and slide into Rack Position 2, select Convection Broil, set temperature to High and set time to 6 minutes.
4. After 2 or 3 minutes, check the pears. The pears should be turned over if the prosciutto is beginning to crisp up and brown. Return to the oven and continue cooking.
5. When cooking is complete, remove from the oven. Drizzle the pears with the balsamic vinegar and serve warm.

309.Garlic Herb Tomatoes

Servings: 4
Cooking Time: 45 Minutes
Ingredients:
- 10 medium-sized tomatoes
- 10 garlic cloves
- Bread crumbs
- Thyme
- Sage
- Oregano

Directions:
1. Start by finely chopping garlic and herbs.
2. Cut tomatoes in half and place cut-side up on a baking sheet lined with parchment paper.
3. Pour garlic and herb mixture over tomatoes.
4. Roast at 350°F for 30 minutes in toaster oven.
5. Top with bread crumbs and roast another 15 minutes.

Nutrition Info: Calories: 103, Sodium: 68 mg, Dietary Fiber: 5.4 g, Total Fat: 1.3 g, Total Carbs: 21.4 g, Protein: 4.4 g.

310.Whole Chicken With Bbq Sauce

Servings: 3
Cooking Time: 25 Minutes
Ingredients:
- 1 whole small chicken, cut into pieces
- 1 tsp salt
- 1 tsp smoked paprika
- 1 tsp garlic powder
- 1 cup BBQ sauce

Directions:
1. Coat the chicken with salt, paprika, and garlic. Place the chicken pieces skin-side down in the greased baking tray. Cook in the oven for around 15 minutes at 400 F on Bake function until slightly golden. Remove to a plate and brush with barbecue sauce. Return the chicken to the oven skin-side up and cook for 5 minutes at 340 F. Serve with more barbecue sauce.

311.Rosemary Chickpeas

Servings: 4
Cooking Time: 20 Minutes
Ingredients:
- 2 (14.5-ounce) cans chickpeas, rinsed
- 2 tbsp olive oil
- 1 tsp dried rosemary
- ½ tsp dried thyme
- ¼ tsp dried sage
- ¼ tsp salt

Directions:
1. In a bowl, mix together chickpeas, oil, rosemary, thyme, sage, and salt. Transfer to a baking pan. Select Bake function, adjust the temperature to 380 F, and press Start. Cook for 15 minutes.

312.Paprika Curly Potatoes

Servings: 2
Cooking Time: 20 Minutes
Ingredients:
- 2 whole potatoes, spiralized
- 1 tbsp olive oil
- Salt and black pepper to taste
- 1 tsp paprika

Directions:
1. Preheat Breville on AirFry function to 390 F.
2. Place the potatoes in a bowl and coat with oil. Transfer them to the frying basket and place in the oven. Press Start and cook for 15 minutes. Sprinkle with salt and paprika and serve.

313.Poached Fennel

Servings: 3
Cooking Time: 6 Minutes
Ingredients:
- Ground nutmeg
- 1 tablespoon white flour
- 2 cups milk
- Salt, to taste
- 2 big fennel bulbs, sliced

- 2 tablespoons butter

Directions:

1. Put the Instant Pot in Saute mode, add the butter and melt. Add the fennel slices, mix and cook until lightly browned.

2. Add the flour, salt, pepper, nutmeg and milk, mix, cover and cook in the manual for 6 minutes. Relieve the pressure, transfer the fennel to the dishes and serve.

Nutrition Info: Calories: 140, Fat: 5, Fiber: 4.7, Carbohydrate: 12, Proteins: 4.4

314.Coriander Artichokes(1)

Servings: 4
Cooking Time: 20 Minutes
Ingredients:

- 12 oz. artichoke hearts
- 1 tbsp. lemon juice
- 1 tsp. coriander, ground
- ½ tsp. cumin seeds
- ½ tsp. olive oil
- Salt and black pepper to taste.

Directions:

1. In a pan that fits your air fryer, mix all the ingredients, toss, introduce the pan in the fryer and cook at 370°F for 15 minutes

2. Divide the mix between plates and serve as a side dish.

Nutrition Info: Calories: 200; Fat: 7g; Fiber: 2g; Carbs: 5g; Protein: 8g

315.Green Bean Casserole(3)

Servings: 4
Cooking Time: 20 Minutes
Ingredients:

- 1 lb. fresh green beans, edges trimmed
- ½ oz. pork rinds, finely ground
- 1 oz. full-fat cream cheese
- ½ cup heavy whipping cream.
- ¼ cup diced yellow onion
- ½ cup chopped white mushrooms
- ½ cup chicken broth
- 4 tbsp. unsalted butter.
- ¼ tsp. xanthan gum

Directions:

1. In a medium skillet over medium heat, melt the butter. Sauté the onion and mushrooms until they become soft and fragrant, about 3–5 minutes.

2. Add the heavy whipping cream, cream cheese and broth to the pan. Whisk until smooth. Bring to a boil and then reduce to a simmer. Sprinkle the xanthan gum into the pan and remove from heat

3. Chop the green beans into 2-inch pieces and place into a 4-cup round baking dish. Pour the sauce mixture over them and stir until coated. Top the dish with ground pork rinds. Place into the air fryer basket

4. Adjust the temperature to 320 Degrees F and set the timer for 15 minutes. Top will be golden and green beans fork tender when fully cooked. Serve warm.

Nutrition Info: Calories: 267; Protein: 6g; Fiber: 2g; Fat: 24g; Carbs: 7g

316.Spinach And Artichokes Sauté

Servings: 4
Cooking Time: 20 Minutes
Ingredients:

- 10 oz. artichoke hearts; halved
- 2 cups baby spinach
- 3 garlic cloves
- ¼ cup veggie stock
- 2 tsp. lime juice
- Salt and black pepper to taste.

Directions:

1. In a pan that fits your air fryer, mix all the ingredients, toss, introduce in the fryer and cook at 370°F for 15 minutes

2. Divide between plates and serve as a side dish.

Nutrition Info: Calories: 209; Fat: 6g; Fiber: 2g; Carbs: 4g; Protein: 8g

317.Savory Cod Fingers

Servings: 3
Cooking Time: 25 Minutes
Ingredients:

- 2 cups flour
- 1 tsp seafood seasoning
- 2 whole eggs, beaten
- 1 cup cornmeal
- 1 pound cod fillets, cut into fingers
- 2 tbsp milk
- 2 eggs, beaten
- 1 cup breadcrumbs

Directions:

1. Preheat Breville on Air Fryer function to 400 F. In a bowl, mix beaten eggs with milk. In a separate bowl, mix flour, cornmeal, and seafood seasoning. In a third bowl, pour the breadcrumbs.

2. Dip cod fingers in the flour mixture, followed by a dip in the egg mixture and finally coat with breadcrumbs. Place the fingers in the frying basket and Press Start. AirFry for 10 minutes.

318.Blistered Shishito Peppers With Lime Juice

Servings: 3
Cooking Time: 9 Minutes
Ingredients:
- ½ pound (227 g) shishito peppers, rinsed
- Cooking spray
- Sauce:
- 1 tablespoon tamari or shoyu
- 2 teaspoons fresh lime juice
- 2 large garlic cloves, minced

Directions:
1. Spritz the air fryer basket with cooking spray.
2. Place the shishito peppers in the basket and spritz them with cooking spray.
3. Put the air fryer basket on the baking pan and slide into Rack Position 2, select Roast, set temperature to 392ºF (200ºC), and set time to 9 minutes.
4. Meanwhile, whisk together all the ingredients for the sauce in a large bowl. Set aside.
5. After 3 minutes, remove from the oven. Flip the peppers and spritz them with cooking spray. Return to the oven and continue cooking.
6. After another 3 minutes, remove from the oven. Flip the peppers and spray with cooking spray. Return to the oven and continue roasting for 3 minutes more, or until the peppers are blistered and nicely browned.
7. When cooking is complete, remove the peppers from the oven to the bowl of sauce. Toss to coat well and serve immediately.

319.Green Beans And Mushrooms

Servings: 4
Cooking Time: 6 Minutes
Ingredients:
- 1 small yellow onion, peeled and chopped
- 6 ounces bacon, chopped
- Salt and ground black pepper, to taste Balsamic vinegar
- 1-pound fresh green beans, trimmed
- 1 garlic clove, peeled and minced
- 8 ounces mushrooms, sliced

Directions:
1. Place the beans in the Instant Pot, add water to cover them, cover the Instant Pot and cook for 3 minutes in manual configuration.
2. Release the pressure naturally, drain the beans and set aside. Place the Instant Pot in the sauté mode, add the bacon and sauté for 1 to 2 minutes, stirring constantly.
3. Add garlic and onion, mix and cook 2 minutes. Add the mushrooms, mix and cook until tender. Add the drain beans, salt, pepper and a pinch of vinegar, mix, remove from heat, divide between plates and serve.
Nutrition Info: Calories: 120, Fat: 3.7, Fiber: 3.3, Carbohydrate: 7.5, Proteins: 2.4

320.Cinnamon Mixed Nuts

Servings: 4
Cooking Time: 25 Minutes
Ingredients:
- ½ cup pecans
- ½ cup walnuts
- ½ cup almonds
- A pinch cayenne pepper
- 2 tbsp sugar
- 2 tbsp egg whites
- 2 tsp cinnamon

Directions:
1. In a bowl, mix the cayenne pepper, sugar, and cinnamon; set aside. In another bowl, beat the egg whites and mix in the pecans, walnuts,and almonds. Add in the spice mixture and stir well.
2. Lightly grease the frying basket with baking tray. Pour in the nuts mixture. Select Toast function, adjust the temperature to 360 F, and press Start. Toast for 10 minutes, then stir the nuts using a wooden vessel, and toast further for 10 minutes. Pour the nuts in a bowl and let cool.

321.Spicy Broccoli With Hot Sauce

Servings: 6
Cooking Time: 14 Minutes
Ingredients:
- Broccoli:
- 1 medium-sized head broccoli, cut into florets
- 1½ tablespoons olive oil
- 1 teaspoon shallot powder
- 1 teaspoon porcini powder
- ½ teaspoon freshly grated lemon zest
- ½ teaspoon hot paprika
- ½ teaspoon granulated garlic
- $^1/_3$ teaspoon fine sea salt
- $^1/_3$ teaspoon celery seeds
- Hot Sauce:
- ½ cup tomato sauce
- 1 tablespoon balsamic vinegar
- ½ teaspoon ground allspice

Directions:
1. In a mixing bowl, combine all the ingredients for the broccoli and toss to coat. Transfer the broccoli to the air fryer basket.
2. Put the air fryer basket on the baking pan and slide into Rack Position 2, select Air Fry, set

temperature to 360ºF (182ºC), and set time to 14 minutes.

3.   Meanwhile, make the hot sauce by whisking together the tomato sauce, balsamic vinegar, and allspice in a small bowl.

4.   When cooking is complete, remove the broccoli from the oven and serve with the hot sauce.

322.Buttered Corn

Servings: 2
Cooking Time: 20 Minutes
Ingredients:
- 2 corn on the cob
- Salt and freshly ground black pepper, as needed
- 2 tablespoons butter, softened and divided

Directions:
1.   Sprinkle the cobs evenly with salt and black pepper.
2.   Then, rub with 1 tablespoon of butter.
3.   With 1 piece of foil, wrap each cob.
4.   Press "Power Button" of Air Fry Oven and turn the dial to select the "Air Fry" mode.
5.   Press the Time button and again turn the dial to set the cooking time to 20 minutes.
6.   Now push the Temp button and rotate the dial to set the temperature at 320 degrees F.
7.   Press "Start/Pause" button to start.
8.   When the unit beeps to show that it is preheated, open the lid.
9.   Arrange the cobs in "Air Fry Basket" and insert in the oven.
10.   Serve warm.

Nutrition Info: Calories 186 Total Fat 12.2 g Saturated Fat 7.4 g Cholesterol 31 mg Sodium 163 mg Total Carbs 20.1 g Fiber 2.5 g Sugar 3.2g Protein 2.9 g

323.Baked Broccoli

Servings: 6
Cooking Time: 20 Minutes
Ingredients:
- 4 cups broccoli florets
- 3 tbsp olive oil
- 1/2 tsp pepper
- 1/2 tsp garlic powder
- 1 tsp Italian seasoning
- 1 tsp salt

Directions:
1.   Fit the oven with the rack in position
2.   Spread broccoli in baking pan and drizzle with oil and season with garlic powder, Italian seasoning, pepper, and salt.
3.   Set to bake at 400 F for 25 minutes. After 5 minutes place the baking pan in the preheated oven.

4.   Serve and enjoy.

Nutrition Info: Calories 84 Fat 7.4 g Carbohydrates 4.4 g Sugar 1.2 g Protein 1.8 g Cholesterol 1 mg

324.Baked Turnip & Sweet Potato

Servings: 4
Cooking Time: 30 Minutes
Ingredients:
- 1 1/2 lbs sweet potato, sliced 1/4-inch thick
- 2 tbsp olive oil
- 1 lb turnips, sliced 1/4-inch thick
- 1 tbsp thyme, chopped
- 1 tsp paprika
- 1/4 tsp pepper
- 1/2 tsp sea salt

Directions:
1.   Fit the oven with the rack in position
2.   Add sliced sweet potatoes and turnips in a bowl and toss with seasoning and olive oil.
3.   Arrange sliced sweet potatoes and turnips in baking dish.
4.   Set to bake at 425 F for 35 minutes. After 5 minutes place the baking dish in the preheated oven.
5.   Garnish with thyme and serve.

Nutrition Info: Calories 250 Fat 7.4 g Carbohydrates 43.5 g Sugar 15.8 g Protein 4.5 g Cholesterol 0 mg

325.Easy Refried Beans

Servings: 4
Cooking Time: 20 Minutes
Ingredients:
- 1 jalapeño, chopped
- 3 cups pinto beans, soaked for 4 hours and drained
- 1 yellow onion, peeled and cut into halves
- Salt and ground black pepper, to taste
- 2 tablespoons garlic, minced
- 9 cups vegetable stock
- 1/8 teaspoon cumin

Directions:
1.   In the Instant Pot, mix the beans with salt, pepper, stock, onion, jalapeno pepper, garlic and cumin. Stir, cover and cook for 20 minutes in the Bean / Chili setting.
2.   Relieve the pressure naturally, discard the onion halves, filter the grains, transfer them to the blender and reserve the cooking liquid. Mix well, add a little liquid, if necessary, transfer to a bowl and serve.

Nutrition Info: Calories: 100, Fat: 2, Fiber: 5, Carbohydrate: 15, Proteins: 6

326.Amul Cheesy Cabbage Canapes

Servings: 2
Cooking Time: 15 Minutes
Ingredients:
- 1 whole cabbage, washed and cut in rounds
- 1 cube Amul cheese
- ½ carrot, cubed
- ¼ onion, cubed
- ¼ red bell pepper, cubed
- 1 tsp fresh basil, chopped

Directions:
1. Preheat on Air Fry function to 360 F. Using a bowl, mix onion, carrot, bell pepper, and cheese. Toss to coat everything evenly. Add cabbage rounds to the Air fryer baking pan.
2. Top with the veggie mixture and cook for 8 minutes. Garnish with basil and serve.

327.Sausage Mushroom Caps(3)

Servings: 2
Cooking Time: 8 Minutes
Ingredients:
- ½ lb. Italian sausage
- 6 large Portobello mushroom caps
- ¼ cup grated Parmesan cheese.
- ¼ cup chopped onion
- 2 tbsp. blanched finely ground almond flour
- 1 tsp. minced fresh garlic

Directions:
1. Use a spoon to hollow out each mushroom cap, reserving scrapings.
2. In a medium skillet over medium heat, brown the sausage about 10 minutes or until fully cooked and no pink remains. Drain and then add reserved mushroom scrapings, onion, almond flour, Parmesan and garlic.
3. Gently fold ingredients together and continue cooking an additional minute, then remove from heat
4. Evenly spoon the mixture into mushroom caps and place the caps into a 6-inch round pan. Place pan into the air fryer basket
5. Adjust the temperature to 375 Degrees F and set the timer for 8 minutes. When finished cooking, the tops will be browned and bubbling. Serve warm.
Nutrition Info: Calories: 404; Protein: 24.3g; Fiber: 4.5g; Fat: 25.8g; Carbs: 18.2g

328.Cheese Eggplant Boats With Ham & Parsley

Servings: 2
Cooking Time: 20 Minutes
Ingredients:
- 1 eggplant
- 4 ham slices, chopped
- 1 cup shredded mozzarella cheese
- 1 tsp dried parsley
- Salt and black pepper to taste

Directions:
1. Preheat on Bake function to 330 F. Peel the eggplant and cut it lengthwise in half; scoop some of the flesh out. Season with salt and pepper. Divide half of the mozzarella cheese between the eggplant halves and cover with the ham slices. Top with the remaining mozzarella cheese, sprinkle with parsley, and cook for 12 minutes. Serve warm.

329.Classic Cauliflower Hash Browns

Servings: 2
Cooking Time: 20 Minutes
Ingredients:
- 2/3 pound cauliflower, peeled and grated
- 2 eggs, whisked
- 1/4 cup scallions, chopped
- 1 teaspoon fresh garlic, minced
- Sea salt and ground black pepper, to taste
- 1/4 teaspoon ground allspice
- 1/2 teaspoon cinnamon
- 1 tablespoon peanut oil

Directions:
1. Boil cauliflower over medium-low heat until fork-tender, 5 to 7 minutes Drain the water; pat cauliflower dry with a kitchen towel.
2. Now, add the remaining ingredients; stir to combine well.
3. Cook in the preheated Air Fryer at 395 degrees F for 20 minutes. Shake the basket once or twice. Serve with low-carb tomato sauce.
Nutrition Info: 157 Calories; 12g Fat; 3g Carbs; 8g Protein; 6g Sugars; 6g Fiber

330.Spicy Crab Cakes

Servings: 4
Cooking Time: 20 Minutes
Ingredients:
- 1 lb crab meat, shredded
- 2 eggs, beaten
- ½ cup breadcrumbs
- ⅓ cup green onions, finely chopped
- ¼ cup parsley, chopped
- 1 tbsp mayonnaise
- 1 tsp sweet chili sauce
- ½ tsp paprika
- Salt and black pepper to taste

Directions:

1. In a bowl, add meat, eggs, crumbs, green onion, parsley, mayo, chili sauce, paprika, salt and pepper; mix well. Shape into cakes and brush with oil.
2. Arrange them on the frying basket without overcrowding. Select AirFry function, adjust the temperature to 400 F, and press Start. Cook for 10-12 minutes.

331.Gourmet Beef Sticks

Servings: 3
Cooking Time: 10 Minutes + Chilling Time
Ingredients:
- 1 lb ground beef
- 3 tbsp sugar
- A pinch garlic powder
- A pinch chili powder
- Salt to taste
- 1 tsp liquid smoke

Directions:
1. Place the beef, sugar, garlic powder, chili powder, salt and liquid smoke in a bowl. Mix well. Mold out 4 sticks with your hands, place them on a plate, and refrigerate for 30 minutes.
2. Remove and cook in the oven at 350 F for 10 minutes on Bake function. Flip and continue cooking for another 5 minutes until browned.

332.Bbq Full Chicken

Servings: 3
Cooking Time: 50 Minutes
Ingredients:
- 1 (3,5 pounds) whole chicken, cut into pieces
- 1 tsp salt
- 1 tsp smoked paprika
- 1 tsp garlic powder
- 1 cup BBQ sauce

Directions:
1. Mix salt, paprika, and garlic and coat chicken pieces. Place them skin-side down in the toaster oven. Select Bake function, adjust the temperature to 400 F, and press Start. Cook for around 25 minutes until slightly golden.
2. Remove to a plate and brush with some barbecue sauce. Return the chicken to the oven, skin-side up and bake for 15-20 more minutes. Serve with the remaining barbecue sauce.

333.Butternut And Apple Mash

Servings: 4
Cooking Time: 15 Minutes
Ingredients:

- 1 butternut squash, peeled and cut into medium chunks
- 2 apples, cored and sliced
- 1 cup water
- ½ teaspoon apple pie spice
- Salt, to taste
- 2 tablespoons butter, browned
- 1 yellow onion, thinly sliced

Directions:
1. Place the pieces of pumpkin, onion and apple in the steam basket of the Instant Pot, add the water to the Instant Pot, cover and cook for 8 minutes in manual setting.
2. Quickly release the pressure and transfer the pumpkin, onion and apple to a bowl. Smash everything with a potato masher, add salt, apple pie spices and brown butter, mix well and serve hot.
Nutrition Info: Calories: 140, Fat: 2.3, Fiber: 6.5, Carbohydrate: 24, Proteins: 2.5

334.Herb Balsamic Mushrooms

Servings: 6
Cooking Time: 20 Minutes
Ingredients:
- 1 lb button mushrooms, scrubbed and stems trimmed
- 2 tbsp olive oil
- 4 tbsp balsamic vinegar
- 1/2 tsp dried basil
- 1/2 tsp dried oregano
- 3 garlic cloves, crushed
- 1/4 tsp black pepper
- 1 tsp sea salt

Directions:
1. Fit the oven with the rack in position
2. In a large bowl, whisk together vinegar, basil, oregano, garlic, olive oil, pepper, and salt. Stir in mushrooms and let sit for 15 minutes.
3. Spread mushrooms in baking pan.
4. Set to bake at 425 F for 25 minutes. After 5 minutes place the baking pan in the preheated oven.
5. Serve and enjoy.
Nutrition Info: Calories 61 Fat 4.9 g Carbohydrates 3.2 g Sugar 1.4 g Protein 2.5 g Cholesterol 0 mg

335.Pineapple Spareribs

Servings: 4
Cooking Time: 35 Minutes
Ingredients:
- 2 lb cut spareribs
- 7 oz salad dressing
- 1 (5-oz) can pineapple juice
- 2 cups water

- 1 tsp garlic powder
- Salt and black pepper

Directions:
1. Sprinkle the ribs with garlic powder, salt, and pepper. Arrange them on the frying basket. sprinkle with garlic salt. Select AirFry function, adjust the temperature to 400 F, and press Start. Cook for 20-25 minutes until golden brown. Prepare the sauce by combining the salad dressing and the pineapple juice. Serve the ribs drizzled with the sauce.

336.Easy Crunchy Garlic Croutons

Servings: 4
Cooking Time: 20 Minutes
Ingredients:
- 2 cups bread, cubed
- 2 tbsp butter, melted
- Garlic salt and black pepper to taste

Directions:
1. In a bowl, toss the bread cubes with butter, garlic salt, and pepper until well-coated. Place the cubes in the Air Fryer basket and fit in the baking tray. Cook in the oven for 12 minutes at 380 F on Air Fry function or until golden brown and crispy.

337.Crispy Calamari Rings

Servings: 4
Cooking Time: 10 Minutes + Chilling Time
Ingredients:
- 1 lb calamari (squid), cut in rings
- ¼ cup flour
- 2 large beaten eggs
- 1 cup breadcrumbs

Directions:
1. Coat the calamari rings with the flour and dip them in the eggs. Then, dip in the breadcrumbs. Refrigerate for 30 minutes. Remove and arrange on the Air Fryer basket and apply cooking spray. Fit in the baking tray and cook for 9 minutes at 380 F on Air Fry function. Serve with garlic mayo and lemon wedges.

338.Cheesy Chicken Breasts With Marinara Sauce

Servings: 2
Cooking Time: 25 Minutes
Ingredients:
- 2 chicken breasts, beaten into ½ inch thick
- 1 egg, beaten
- ½ cup breadcrumbs
- Salt and black pepper to taste
- 2 tbsp marinara sauce

- 2 tbsp Grana Padano cheese, grated
- 2 mozzarella cheese slices

Directions:
1. Dip the breasts into the egg, then into the crumbs and arrange on the fryer basket. Select AirFry function, adjust the temperature to 400 F, and press Start. Cook for 5 minutes, turn over, and drizzle with marinara sauce, Grana Padano and mozzarella cheeses. Cook for 5 more minutes.

339.Rosemary Roasted Potatoes

Servings: 4
Cooking Time: 20 Minutes
Ingredients:
- 1½ pounds (680 g) small red potatoes, cut into 1-inch cubes
- 2 tablespoons olive oil
- 2 tablespoons minced fresh rosemary
- 1 tablespoon minced garlic
- 1 teaspoon salt, plus additional as needed
- ½ teaspoon freshly ground black pepper, plus additional as needed

Directions:
1. Toss the potato cubes with the olive oil, rosemary, garlic, salt, and pepper in a large bowl until thoroughly coated.
2. Arrange the potato cubes in the air fryer basket in a single layer.
3. Put the air fryer basket on the baking pan and slide into Rack Position 2, select Roast, set temperature to 400ºF (205ºC), and set time to 20 minutes.
4. Stir the potatoes a few times during cooking for even cooking.
5. When cooking is complete, the potatoes should be tender. Remove from the oven to a plate. Taste and add additional salt and pepper as needed.

340.French Fries

Servings: 4
Cooking Time: 10 Minutes
Ingredients:
- ¼ teaspoon baking soda Oil for frying
- Salt, to taste
- 8 medium potatoes, peeled, cut into medium matchsticks, and patted dry
- 1 cup water

Directions:
1. Put the water in the Instant Pot, add the salt and baking soda and mix. Place the potatoes in the steam basket and place them in the Instant Pot, cover and cook with manual adjustment for 3 minutes.

2. Release the pressure naturally, remove the chips from the Instant Pot and place them in a bowl. Heat a pan with enough oil over medium-high heat, add the potatoes, spread and cook until they are golden brown.

3. Transfer the potatoes to the paper towels to drain the excess fat and place them in a bowl. Salt, mix well and serve.

Nutrition Info: Calories: 300, Fat: 10, Fiber: 3.7, Carbohydrate: 41, Proteins: 3.4

341.Spicy Pumpkin-ham Fritters

Servings: 4
Cooking Time: 10 Minutes
Ingredients:
- 1 oz ham, chopped
- 1 cup dry pancake mix
- 1 egg
- 2 tbsp canned puree pumpkin
- 1 oz cheddar, shredded
- ½ tsp chili powder
- 3 tbsp of flour
- 1 oz beer
- 2 tbsp scallions, chopped

Directions:
1. Preheat on Air Fry function to 370 F. In a bowl, combine the pancake mix and chili powder. Mix in the egg, puree pumpkin, beer, shredded cheddar, ham and scallions. Form balls and roll them in the flour.

2. Arrange the balls into the basket and fit in the baking tray. Cook for 8 minutes. Drain on paper towel before serving.

342.Pumpkin Fritters With Ham & Cheese

Servings: 4
Cooking Time: 10 Minutes
Ingredients:
- ½ cup ham, chopped
- 1 cup dry pancake mix
- 1 egg
- 2 tbsp canned puree pumpkin
- 1 oz cheddar, shredded
- ½ tsp chili powder
- 3 tbsp of flour
- ½ cup beer
- 2 tbsp scallions, chopped

Directions:
1. Preheat Breville on AirFry function to 370 F. In a bowl, combine the pancake mix and chili powder. Mix in the egg, puree pumpkin, beer, cheddar cheese, ham, and scallions. Form balls and roll them in the flour. Arrange the balls into the basket. Press Start and cook for 12 minutes.

MEAT RECIPES

343.Juicy Chicken Patties

Servings: 4
Cooking Time: 25 Minutes
Ingredients:
- 1 egg
- 1 lb ground chicken
- 1 tsp garlic, minced
- 1/2 cup onion, minced
- 3/4 cup breadcrumbs
- 1/2 cup mozzarella cheese, grated cheese
- 1 cup carrot, grated
- 1 cup cauliflower, grated
- 1/8 tsp pepper
- 3/4 tsp salt

Directions:
1. Fit the oven with the rack in position
2. Add all ingredients into the mixing bowl and mix until well combined.
3. Make 4 equal shapes of patties from meat mixture and place onto the parchment-lined baking pan.
4. Set to bake at 400 F for 30 minutes. After 5 minutes place the baking pan in the preheated oven.
5. Serve and enjoy.
Nutrition Info: Calories 346 Fat 11.2 g Carbohydrates 20.4 g Sugar 3.9 g Protein 38.8 g Cholesterol 144 mg

344.White Wine Chicken Wings

Servings: 2
Cooking Time: 30 Minutes
Ingredients:
- 8 chicken wings
- ½ tbsp sugar
- 2 tbsp cornflour
- ½ tbsp white wine
- 1 tbsp fresh ginger, grated
- ½ tbsp olive oil

Directions:
1. In a bowl, mix olive oil, ginger, white wine, and sugar. Add in the chicken wings and toss to coat. Roll up in the flour. Place the chicken in the frying basket and press Start. Cook for 20 minutes until crispy on the outside at 320 F on AirFry function. Serve warm.

345.Air Fried Golden Wasabi Spam

Servings: 3
Cooking Time: 12 Minutes
Ingredients:
- $^2/_3$ cup all-purpose flour
- 2 large eggs
- 1½ tablespoons wasabi paste
- 2 cups panko bread crumbs
- 6 ½-inch-thick spam slices
- Cooking spray

Directions:
1. Spritz the air fryer basket with cooking spray.
2. Pour the flour in a shallow plate. Whisk the eggs with wasabi in a large bowl. Pour the panko in a separate shallow plate.
3. Dredge the spam slices in the flour first, then dunk in the egg mixture, and then roll the spam over the panko to coat well. Shake the excess off.
4. Arrange the spam slices in the pan and spritz with cooking spray.
5. Put the air fryer basket on the baking pan and slide into Rack Position 2, select Air Fry, set temperature to 400ºF (205ºC) and set time to 12 minutes.
6. Flip the spam slices halfway through.
7. When cooking is complete, the spam slices should be golden and crispy.
8. Serve immediately.

346.Chicken Madeira

Ingredients:
- 2 cups Madeira wine
- 2 cups beef broth
- ½ cup shredded Mozzarella cheese
- 4 boneless, skinless chicken breasts
- 1 Tbsp salt
- Salt and freshly ground black pepper, to taste
- 6 cups water
- ½ lb. asparagus, trimmed
- 2 Tbsp extra-virgin olive oil
- 2 Tbsp chopped fresh parsley

Directions:
1. Lay the chicken breasts on a cutting board, and cover each with a piece of plastic wrap. Use a mallet or a small, heavy frying pan to pound them to ¼ inch thick. Discard the plastic wrap and season with salt and pepper on both sides of the chicken.
2. Fill oven with the water, bring to a boil, and add the salt.
3. Add the asparagus and boil, uncovered, until crisp, tender, and bright green, 2 to 3 minutes. Remove immediately and set aside. Pour out the water.
4. In oven over medium heat, heat the olive oil. Cook the chicken for 4 to 5 minutes on each side. Remove and set aside.

5. Add the Madeira wine and beef broth. Bring to a boil, reduce to a simmer, and cook for 10 to 12 minutes.
6. Return the chicken to the pot, turning it to coat in the sauce.
7. Lay the asparagus and cheese on top of the chicken. Then transfer oven to the oven broiler and broil for 3 to 4 minutes. Garnish with the parsley, if using, and serve.

347.Baked Fajita Chicken

Servings: 4
Cooking Time: 35 Minutes
Ingredients:
- 4 chicken breasts, sliced
- 2 cups cheddar cheese, shredded
- 2 bell peppers, sliced
- 1 oz fajita seasoning
- 1/3 cup salsa
- 8 oz cream cheese, softened

Directions:
1. Fit the oven with the rack in position
2. Place chicken into the greased 9*13-inch baking dish.
3. Mix together salsa, cream cheese, and fajita seasoning and pour over chicken.
4. Spread sliced bell peppers on top of chicken. Sprinkle shredded cheese on top.
5. Set to bake at 375 F for 40 minutes. After 5 minutes place the baking dish in the preheated oven.
6. Serve and enjoy.
Nutrition Info: Calories 754 Fat 49.5 g Carbohydrates 252 g Sugar 4.1 g Protein 61.5 g Cholesterol 252 mg

348.Festive Stuffed Pork Chops

Servings: 4
Cooking Time: 40 Minutes
Ingredients:
- 4 pork chops
- Salt and black pepper to taste
- 4 cups stuffing mix
- 2 tbsp olive oil
- 4 garlic cloves, minced
- 2 tbsp fresh sage leaves, chopped

Directions:
1. Cut a hole in pork chops and fill chops with stuffing mix. In a bowl, mix sage, garlic, oil, salt, and pepper. Rub the chops with the marinade and let sit for 10 minutes.
2. Preheat Breville on Bake function to 380 F. Put the chops in a baking tray and place in the oven. Press Start and cook for 25 minutes. Serve and enjoy!

349.Honey Chili Chicken

Ingredients:
- 1 capsicum (Cut in to long pieces)
- 2 small onions. Cut them into halves
- 1 ½ tsp. ginger garlic paste
- ½ tbsp. red chili sauce
- 2 tbsp. tomato ketchup
- 1 ½ tbsp. sweet chili sauce
- 2 tsp. soya sauce
- 2 tsp. vinegar
- 1-2 tbsp. honey
- 1 lb. chicken (Cut the chicken into slices)
- 2 ½ tsp. ginger-garlic paste
- 1 tsp. red chili sauce
- ¼ tsp. salt
- ¼ tsp. red chili powder/black pepper
- A few drops of edible orange food coloring
- 2 tbsp. olive oil
- A pinch of black pepper
- 2 tsp. red chili flakes

Directions:
1. Create the mix for the chicken Oregano Fingers and coat the chicken well with it.
2. Pre heat the oven at 250 Fahrenheit for 5 minutes or so. Open the basket of the Fryer. Place the Oregano Fingers inside the basket. Now let the fryer stay at 290 Fahrenheit for another 20 minutes. Keep tossing the Oregano Fingers periodically through the cook to get a uniform cook.
3. Add the ingredients to the sauce and cook it with the vegetables till it thickens. Add the chicken Oregano Fingers to the sauce and cook till the flavors have blended.

350.Garlic Infused Roast Beef

Servings: 10
Cooking Time: 75 Minutes
Ingredients:
- 3 lb. beef roast, room temperature
- 4 cloves garlic, cut in thin slivers
- Olive oil spray,
- 1 tsp salt
- 1 tsp pepper
- 2 tsp rosemary

Directions:
1. Trim off the fat from the roast. Use a sharp knife to pierce the roast in intervals, ½-inch deep. Insert garlic sliver in holes, pushing into the meat.
2. Lightly spray the beef with oil and season with salt, pepper, and rosemary.
3. Place the baking pan in position 1 of the oven. Set to convection bake on 325°F for 60 minutes.

4. Spray the fryer basket with oil and place roast in it. Once the oven has preheated for 5 minutes, place the basket on the pan. Cook 60 minutes, or until beef reaches desired doneness.
5. Remove from oven and let rest 10 minutes. Slice thinly and serve.
Nutrition Info: Calories 265, Total Fat 13g, Saturated Fat 5g, Total Carbs 1g, Net Carbs 1g, Protein 36g, Sugar 0g, Fiber 0g, Sodium 342mg, Potassium 478mg, Phosphorus 288mg

351.Chicken Wings With Chili-lime Sauce

Servings: 2
Cooking Time: 25 Minutes
Ingredients:
- 10 chicken wings
- 2 tbsp hot chili sauce
- ½ tbsp lime juice
- Salt and black pepper to taste

Directions:
1. Preheat Breville on AirFry function to 350 F. Mix lime juice and chili sauce. Toss in the chicken wings. Transfer them to the basket and press Start. Cook for 25 minutes. Serve.

352.Chicken Wings With Honey & Cashew Cream

Servings: 4
Cooking Time: 25 Minutes
Ingredients:
- 2 lb chicken wings
- 1 tbsp fresh cilantro, chopped
- Salt and black pepper to taste
- 1 tbsp cashews cream
- 1 garlic clove, minced
- 1 tbsp plain yogurt
- 2 tbsp honey
- ½ tbsp white wine vinegar
- ½ tbsp ginger, minced
- ½ tbsp garlic chili sauce

Directions:
1. Preheat Breville on AirFry function to 360 F. Season the wings with salt and black pepper, place them in a baking dish. Press Start and cook for 15 minutes. In a bowl, mix the remaining ingredients. Top the chicken with sauce and cook for 5 more minutes. Serve warm.

353.Turkey And Cauliflower Meatloaf

Servings: 6
Cooking Time: 50 Minutes
Ingredients:

- 2 pounds (907 g) lean ground turkey
- 1^1/$_3$ cups riced cauliflower
- 2 large eggs, lightly beaten
- ¼ cup almond flour
- ^{2}/$_3$ cup chopped yellow or white onion
- 1 teaspoon ground dried turmeric
- 1 teaspoon ground cumin
- 1 teaspoon ground coriander
- 1 tablespoon minced garlic
- 1 teaspoon salt
- 1 teaspoon ground black pepper
- Cooking spray

Directions:
1. Spritz the baking pan with cooking spray.
2. Combine all the ingredients in a large bowl. Stir to mix well. Pour half of the mixture in the prepared pan and press with a spatula to coat the bottom evenly. Spritz the mixture with cooking spray.
3. Slide the baking pan into Rack Position 1, select Convection Bake, set temperature to 350ºF (180ºC) and set time to 25 minutes.
4. When cooking is complete, the meat should be well browned and the internal temperature should reach at least 165ºF (74ºC).
5. Remove the pan from the oven and serve immediately.

354.Air Fryer Herb Pork Chops

Servings: 4
Cooking Time: 15 Minutes
Ingredients:
- 4 pork chops
- 2 tsp oregano
- 2 tsp thyme
- 2 tsp sage
- 1 tsp garlic powder
- 1 tsp paprika
- 1 tsp rosemary
- Pepper
- Salt

Directions:
1. Fit the oven with the rack in position 2.
2. Line the air fryer basket with parchment paper.
3. Mix garlic powder, paprika, rosemary, oregano, thyme, sage, pepper, and salt and rub over pork chops.
4. Place pork chops in the air fryer basket then place an air fryer basket in the baking pan.
5. Place a baking pan on the oven rack. Set to air fry at 360 F for 15 minutes.
6. Serve and enjoy.
Nutrition Info: Calories 266 Fat 20.2 g Carbohydrates 2 g Sugar 0.3 g Protein 18.4 g Cholesterol 69 mg

355.Air Fried Beef Satay With Peanut Dipping Sauce

Servings: 4
Cooking Time: 5 Minutes
Ingredients:
- 8 ounces (227 g) London broil, sliced into 8 strips
- 2 teaspoons curry powder
- ½ teaspoon kosher salt
- Cooking spray
- Peanut Dipping sauce:
- 2 tablespoons creamy peanut butter
- 1 tablespoon reduced-sodium soy sauce
- 2 teaspoons rice vinegar
- 1 teaspoon honey
- 1 teaspoon grated ginger
- Special Equipment:
- 4 bamboo skewers, cut into halves and soaked in water for 20 minutes to keep them from burning while cooking

Directions:
1. Spritz the air fryer basket with cooking spray.
2. In a bowl, place the London broil strips and sprinkle with the curry powder and kosher salt to season. Thread the strips onto the soaked skewers.
3. Arrange the skewers in the prepared basket and spritz with cooking spray.
4. Put the air fryer basket on the baking pan and slide into Rack Position 2, select Air Fry, set temperature to 360ºF (182ºC) and set time to 5 minutes.
5. Flip the beef halfway through the cooking time.
6. When cooking is complete, the beef should be well browned.
7. In the meantime, stir together the peanut butter, soy sauce, rice vinegar, honey, and ginger in a bowl to make the dipping sauce.
8. Transfer the beef to the serving dishes and let rest for 5 minutes. Serve with the peanut dipping sauce on the side.

356.Teriyaki Pork Ribs In Tomato Sauce

Servings: 4
Cooking Time: 20 Minutes
Ingredients:
- 1 pound pork ribs
- Salt and black pepper to taste
- 1 tbsp sugar
- 1 tsp ginger juice
- 1 tsp five-spice powder
- 1 tbsp teriyaki sauce
- 1 tbsp soy sauce
- 1 garlic clove, minced
- 2 tbsp honey
- 1 tbsp water
- 1 tbsp tomato sauce

Directions:
1. In a bowl, mix pepper, sugar, five-spice powder, salt, ginger juice, and teriyaki sauce. Add in the pork ribs and let marinate for 2 hours.
2. Preheat Breville on Bake function to 380 F. Put the marinated pork ribs in a baking tray and place in the oven. Press Start and cook for 8 minutes.
3. In a pan over medium heat, mix soy sauce, garlic, honey, water, and tomato sauce. Stir and cook for 2-3 minutes until the sauce thickens. Pour the sauce over the pork ribs and serve.

357.Spicy Meatballs

Servings: 4
Cooking Time: 30 Minutes
Ingredients:
- 1 lb ground beef
- 4 oz cream cheese
- 1 tsp dried basil
- 2 tbsp Worcestershire sauce
- 1/3 cup milk
- 1/2 cup cheddar cheese, shredded
- 3/4 cup breadcrumbs
- 2 jalapenos, minced
- 1/2 onion, minced
- 1 tsp salt

Directions:
1. Fit the oven with the rack in position
2. Add all ingredients into the mixing bowl and mix until well combined.
3. Make small balls from the meat mixture and place it into the parchment-lined baking pan.
4. Set to bake at 400 F for 35 minutes. After 5 minutes place the baking pan in the preheated oven.
5. Serve and enjoy.

Nutrition Info: Calories 472 Fat 23.2 g Carbohydrates 19.7 g Sugar 4.6 g Protein 43.7 g Cholesterol 149 mg

358.Herby Turkey Balls

Servings: 2
Cooking Time: 20 Minutes
Ingredients:
- ½ lb ground turkey
- 1 egg, beaten
- 1 cup breadcrumbs
- 1 tbsp dried thyme
- ½ tbsp dried parsley
- Salt and black pepper to taste

Directions:
1. Preheat Breville on AirFry function to 350 F. In a bowl, place ground turkey, thyme, parsley, salt, and pepper. Mix well and shape the mixture into balls. Dip in breadcrumbs, then in the egg, and finally in the breadcrumbs again. Place the nuggets in the basket and cook for 15 minutes.

359. Pork Burger Patties

Servings: 6
Cooking Time: 35 Minutes
Ingredients:
- 2 lbs ground pork
- 1 egg, lightly beaten
- 1 onion, minced
- 1 carrot, minced
- 1/2 cup breadcrumbs
- 1 tsp garlic powder
- 1 tsp paprika
- Pepper
- Salt

Directions:
1. Fit the oven with the rack in position
2. Add all ingredients into the mixing bowl and mix until well combined.
3. Make small patties from the meat mixture and place it into the baking pan.
4. Set to bake at 375 F for 40 minutes. After 5 minutes place the baking pan in the preheated oven.
5. Serve and enjoy.
Nutrition Info: Calories 276 Fat 6.6 g Carbohydrates 9.8 g Sugar 2.1 g Protein 42.1 g Cholesterol 138 mg

360. Glazed Duck With Cherry Sauce

Servings: 12
Cooking Time: 32 Minutes
Ingredients:
- 1 whole duck (about 5 pounds / 2.3 kg in total), split in half, back and rib bones removed, fat trimmed
- 1 teaspoon olive oil
- Salt and freshly ground black pepper, to taste
- Cherry Sauce:
- 1 tablespoon butter
- 1 shallot, minced
- ½ cup sherry
- 1 cup chicken stock
- 1 teaspoon white wine vinegar
- ¾ cup cherry preserves
- 1 teaspoon fresh thyme leaves
- Salt and freshly ground black pepper, to taste

Directions:

1. On a clean work surface, rub the duck with olive oil, then sprinkle with salt and ground black pepper to season.
2. Place the duck in the air fryer basket, breast side up.
3. Put the air fryer basket on the baking pan and slide into Rack Position 2, select Air Fry, set temperature to 400ºF (205ºC) and set time to 25 minutes.
4. Flip the ducks halfway through the cooking time.
5. Meanwhile, make the cherry sauce: Heat the butter in a skillet over medium-high heat or until melted.
6. Add the shallot and sauté for 5 minutes or until lightly browned.
7. Add the sherry and simmer for 6 minutes or until it reduces in half.
8. Add the chicken stick, white wine vinegar, and cherry preserves. Stir to combine well. Simmer for 6 more minutes or until thickened.
9. Fold in the thyme leaves and sprinkle with salt and ground black pepper. Stir to mix well.
10. When the cooking of the duck is complete, glaze the duck with a quarter of the cherry sauce, then air fry for another 4 minutes.
11. Flip the duck and glaze with another quarter of the cherry sauce. Air fry for an additional 3 minutes.
12. Transfer the duck on a large plate and serve with remaining cherry sauce.

361. Stuffed Pork Chops

Servings: 4
Cooking Time: 35 Minutes
Ingredients:
- 4 pork chops, boneless and thick-cut
- 2 tbsp olives, chopped
- 3 tbsp sun-dried tomatoes, chopped
- 1/2 cup goat cheese, crumbled
- 3 garlic cloves, minced
- 2 tbsp fresh parsley, chopped

Directions:
1. Fit the oven with the rack in position
2. In a bowl, combine together cheese, garlic, parsley, olives, and sun-dried tomatoes.
3. Stuff cheese mixture all the pork chops.
4. Season pork chops with pepper and salt and place in baking pan.
5. Set to bake at 375 F for 40 minutes. After 5 minutes place the baking pan in the preheated oven.
6. Serve and enjoy.
Nutrition Info: Calories 295 Fat 22.6 g Carbohydrates 1.6 g Sugar 0.4 g Protein 20.2 g Cholesterol 75 mg

362.Cripsy Crusted Pork Chops

Servings: 4
Cooking Time: 40 Minutes
Ingredients:
- 4 pork chops, boneless
- 1 cup parmesan cheese
- 1 tbsp olive oil
- 1 tsp garlic powder
- 1 cup breadcrumbs
- 1/2 tsp Italian seasoning
- Pepper
- Salt

Directions:
1. Fit the oven with the rack in position
2. In a shallow dish, mix breadcrumbs, parmesan cheese, Italian seasoning, garlic powder, pepper, and salt.
3. Brush pork chops with oil and coat with breadcrumb mixture.
4. Place coated pork chops in a baking pan.
5. Set to bake at 350 F for 45 minutes. After 5 minutes place the baking pan in the preheated oven.
6. Serve and enjoy.

Nutrition Info: Calories 469 Fat 29.8 g Carbohydrates 20.8 g Sugar 1.9 g Protein 28.9 g Cholesterol 85 mg

363.Bacon Broccoli Chicken

Servings: 4
Cooking Time: 30 Minutes
Ingredients:
- 4 chicken breasts, sliced in half
- 1/3 cup mozzarella cheese, shredded
- 1 cup cheddar cheese, shredded
- 1/2 cup ranch dressing
- 6 bacon slices, cooked & chopped
- 2 cups broccoli florets, chopped

Directions:
1. Fit the oven with the rack in position
2. Place chicken into the greased casserole dish.
3. Add ranch dressing, bacon, and broccoli on top of chicken.
4. Sprinkle cheddar cheese and mozzarella cheese on top of chicken.
5. Set to bake at 375 F for 35 minutes. After 5 minutes place the casserole dish in the preheated oven.
6. Serve and enjoy.

Nutrition Info: Calories 577 Fat 32.8 g Carbohydrates 5.5 g Sugar 1.7 g Protein 62.2 g Cholesterol 192 mg

364.Delicious Turkey Cutlets

Servings: 4
Cooking Time: 25 Minutes
Ingredients:
- 1 egg
- 1 1/2 lbs turkey cutlets
- 1/2 tsp garlic powder
- 1/2 tsp onion powder
- 1/2 tsp dried parsley
- 1/4 cup parmesan cheese, grated
- 1/2 cup almond flour
- 1/4 tsp pepper
- 1/2 tsp salt

Directions:
1. Fit the oven with the rack in position
2. Add egg in a small bowl and whisk well.
3. In a shallow dish, mix almond flour, parmesan cheese, parsley, onion powder, garlic powder, pepper, and salt.
4. Dip turkey cutlet into the egg and coat with almond flour mixture.
5. Place coated turkey cutlets into the baking pan.
6. Set to bake at 350 F for 30 minutes. After 5 minutes place the baking pan in the preheated oven.
7. Serve and enjoy.

Nutrition Info: Calories 346 Fat 12.6 g Carbohydrates 1.6 g Sugar 0.4 g Protein 53.9 g Cholesterol 174 mg

365.Fried Chicken Livers

Servings: 4
Cooking Time: 10 Minutes
Ingredients:
- 1 pound chicken livers
- 1 cup flour
- 1/2 cup cornmeal
- 2 teaspoons your favorite seasoning blend
- 3 eggs
- 2 tablespoons milk

Directions:
1. Preparing the Ingredients. Clean and rinse the livers, pat dry.
2. Beat eggs in a shallow bowl and mix in milk.
3. In another bowl combine flour, cornmeal, and seasoning, mixing until even.
4. Dip the livers in the egg mix, then toss them in the flour mix.
5. Air Frying. Air-fry at 375 degrees for 10 minutes using your air fryer oven. Toss at least once halfway through.

Nutrition Info: CALORIES: 409; FAT: 11G; PROTEIN:36G; FIBER:2G

366.Chuck And Sausage Subs

Servings: 4
Cooking Time: 24 Minutes
Ingredients:
- 1 large egg
- ¼ cup whole milk
- 24 saltines, crushed but not pulverized
- 1 pound (454 g) ground chuck
- 1 pound (454 g) Italian sausage, casings removed
- 4 tablespoons grated Parmesan cheese, divided
- 1 teaspoon kosher salt
- 4 sub rolls, split
- 1 cup Marinara sauce
- ¾ cup shredded Mozzarella cheese

Directions:
1. In a large bowl, whisk the egg into the milk, then stir in the crackers. Let sit for 5 minutes to hydrate.
2. With your hands, break the ground chuck and sausage into the milk mixture, alternating beef and sausage. When you've added half of the meat, sprinkle 2 tablespoons of the grated Parmesan and the salt over it, then continue breaking up the meat until it's all in the bowl. Gently mix everything together. Try not to overwork the meat, but get it all combined.
3. Form the mixture into balls about the size of a golf ball. You should get about 24 meatballs. Flatten the balls slightly to prevent them from rolling, then place them in the baking pan, about 2 inches apart.
4. Slide the baking pan into Rack Position 2, select Roast, set temperature to 400ºF (205ºC), and set time to 20 minutes.
5. After 10 minutes, remove from the oven and turn over the meatballs. Return to the oven and continue cooking.
6. When cooking is complete, remove from the oven. Place the meatballs on a rack. Wipe off the baking pan.
7. Open the rolls, cut-side up, on the baking pan. Place 3 to 4 meatballs on the base of each roll, and top each sandwich with ¼ cup of marinara sauce. Divide the Mozzarella among the top halves of the buns and sprinkle the remaining Parmesan cheese over the Mozzarella.
8. Select Convection Broil, set temperature to High, and set time to 4 minutes.
9. Check the sandwiches after 2 minutes; the Mozzarella cheese should be melted and bubbling slightly.
10. When cooking is complete, remove from the oven. Close the sandwiches and serve.

367.Yakitori

Servings: 4
Cooking Time: 15 Minutes
Ingredients:
- ½ cup mirin
- ¼ cup dry white wine
- ½ cup soy sauce
- 1 tablespoon light brown sugar
- 1½ pounds (680 g) boneless, skinless chicken thighs, cut into 1½-inch pieces, fat trimmed
- 4 medium scallions, trimmed, cut into 1½-inch pieces
- Cooking spray

Directions:
1. Special Equipment:
2. (4-inch) bamboo skewers, soaked in water for at least 30 minutes
3. Combine the mirin, dry white wine, soy sauce, and brown sugar in a saucepan. Bring to a boil over medium heat. Keep stirring.
4. Boil for another 2 minutes or until it has a thick consistency. Turn off the heat.
5. Spritz the air fryer basket with cooking spray.
6. Run the bamboo skewers through the chicken pieces and scallions alternatively.
7. Arrange the skewers in the basket, then brush with mirin mixture on both sides. Spritz with cooking spray.
8. Put the air fryer basket on the baking pan and slide into Rack Position 2, select Air Fry, set temperature to 400ºF (205ºC) and set time to 10 minutes.
9. Flip the skewers halfway through.
10. When cooking is complete, the chicken and scallions should be glossy.
11. Serve immediately.

368.Cheesy Pork Chops

Servings: 4
Cooking Time: 40 Minutes
Ingredients:
- 4 pork chops
- 1/2 tsp garlic powder
- 1/2 tsp pepper
- 1/2 tsp dried parsley
- 1/4 tsp paprika
- 1/4 cup Italian seasoned breadcrumbs
- 1/2 cup parmesan cheese, grated
- 1 tbsp olive oil
- Salt

Directions:
1. Fit the oven with the rack in position
2. In a shallow dish, mix cheese, paprika, breadcrumbs, parsley, pepper, garlic powder, and salt.
3. Brush pork chops with oil and coat with parmesan cheese.

4. Place coated pork chops into the baking dish.
5. Set to bake at 350 F for 45 minutes. After 5 minutes place the baking dish in the preheated oven.
6. Serve and enjoy.
Nutrition Info: Calories 353 Fat 26.2 g Carbohydrates 6 g Sugar 0.5 g Protein 22.8 g Cholesterol 77 mg

369.Italian Chicken Casserole

Servings: 4
Cooking Time: 30 Minutes
Ingredients:
*   Nonstick cooking spray.
*   2 tbsp. olive oil
*   1 cup chicken breasts, boneless, skinless & cut in 1-inch pieces
*   2/3 onion, chopped
*   1 clove garlic, chopped fine
*   1 cup elbow macaroni, cook according to pkg. directions, drain
*   14 ½ oz. tomatoes, diced
*   1 ¼ cups mozzarella cheese, grated
*   ¼ cup fresh parsley, chopped
*   ½ tsp salt
*   ¼ tsp pepper
*   ¼ cup bread crumbs
*   1/3 cup parmesan cheese, grated
*   2 tbsp. butter, melted
Directions:
1. Place the rack in position 1 of the oven. Spray an 8-inch square baking dish with cooking spray.
2. Heat oil in a medium skillet over medium heat. Add chicken and cook 3 minutes, stirring occasionally.
3. And onions and garlic and cook until onions are soft and chicken is no longer pink, about 5 minutes.
4. In a large bowl, combine pasta and chicken. Stir in tomatoes with their juice, mozzarella cheese, parsley, salt, and pepper. Transfer to prepared baking dish.
5. Set oven to bake on 400°F for 35 minutes.
6. In a small bowl, stir together bread crumbs, parmesan cheese, and butter. Sprinkle on top of casserole.
7. Once oven has preheated for 5 minutes, add casserole and bake 30 minutes until top is golden brown. Serve.
Nutrition Info: Calories 427, Total Fat 17g, Saturated Fat 6g, Total Carbs 36g, Net Carbs 32g, Protein 30g, Sugar 7g, Fiber 4g, Sodium 1011mg, Potassium 560mg, Phosphorus 463mg

370.Cheesy Baked Burger Patties

Servings: 6
Cooking Time: 15 Minutes
Ingredients:
*   2 lbs ground beef
*   1 tsp onion powder
*   1 tsp garlic powder
*   1/2 cup mozzarella cheese, shredded
*   1/2 cup cheddar cheese, shredded
*   Pepper
*   Salt
Directions:
1. Fit the oven with the rack in position
2. Add all ingredients into the large bowl and mix until well combined.
3. Make patties from the meat mixture and place it into the baking pan.
4. Set to bake at 400 F for 20 minutes. After 5 minutes place the baking pan in the preheated oven.
5. Serve and enjoy.
Nutrition Info: Calories 329 Fat 13 g Carbohydrates 0.9 g Sugar 0.3 g Protein 49 g Cholesterol 146 mg

371.Barbecue Chicken And Coleslaw Tostadas

Servings: 4 Tostadas
Cooking Time: 10 Minutes
Ingredients:
*   Coleslaw:
*   ¼ cup sour cream
*   ¼ small green cabbage, finely chopped
*   ½ tablespoon white vinegar
*   ½ teaspoon garlic powder
*   ½ teaspoon salt
*   ¼ teaspoon ground black pepper
*   Tostadas:
*   2 cups pulled rotisserie chicken
*   ½ cup barbecue sauce
*   4 corn tortillas
*   ½ cup shredded Mozzarella cheese
*   Cooking spray
Directions:
1. Make the Coleslaw:
2. Combine the ingredients for the coleslaw in a large bowl. Toss to mix well.
3. Refrigerate until ready to serve.
4. Make the Tostadas:
5. Spritz the air fryer basket with cooking spray.
6. Toss the chicken with barbecue sauce in a separate large bowl to combine well. Set aside.
7. Place one tortilla in the basket and spritz with cooking spray.
8. Put the air fryer basket on the baking pan and slide into Rack Position 2, select Air Fry, set

temperature to 370ºF (188ºC) and set time to 10 minutes.

9. Flip the tortilla and spread the barbecue chicken and cheese over halfway through.

10. When cooking is complete, the tortilla should be browned and the cheese should be melted.

11. Serve the tostadas with coleslaw on top.

372.Baked Pork Tenderloin

Servings: 6
Cooking Time: 35 Minutes
Ingredients:
- 2 lbs pork tenderloin
- 3 garlic cloves, chopped
- Pepper
- Salt
- For the spice mix:
- 1/4 tsp chili powder
- 1/4 tsp cayenne
- 1 tsp cinnamon
- 1 tsp cumin
- 1 tsp coriander
- 1 tsp oregano
- 1/4 tsp cloves

Directions:
1. Fit the oven with the rack in position
2. In a small bowl, mix all spice ingredients and set aside.
3. Using a sharp knife make slits on pork tenderloin and insert garlic into each slit.
4. Rub spice mixture over pork tenderloin.
5. Place pork tenderloin in baking pan.
6. Set to bake at 375 F for 40 minutes. After 5 minutes place the baking pan in the preheated oven.
7. Slice and serve.

Nutrition Info: Calories 222 Fat 5.5 g Carbohydrates 1.3 g Sugar 0.1 g Protein 39.8 g Cholesterol 110 mg

373.Easy Smothered Chicken

Servings: 4
Cooking Time: 55 Minutes
Ingredients:
- 4 chicken breasts
- 1/2 tsp garlic powder
- 1 tsp dried basil
- 1 tsp dried oregano
- 1 tbsp cornstarch
- 3/4 cup parmesan cheese, grated
- 1 cup sour cream
- 4 mozzarella cheese slices
- 1/4 tsp pepper
- 1/2 tsp salt

Directions:

1. Fit the oven with the rack in position
2. Place chicken breasts into the baking dish and top with mozzarella cheese slices.
3. In a bowl, mix sour cream, parmesan cheese, cornstarch, oregano, basil, garlic powder, pepper, and salt.
4. Pour sour cream mixture over chicken.
5. Set to bake at 375 F for 60 minutes. After 5 minutes place the baking dish in the preheated oven.
6. Serve and enjoy.

Nutrition Info: Calories 545 Fat 31.5 g Carbohydrates 6.5 g Sugar 0.2 g Protein 57.2 g Cholesterol 182 mg

374.Meatballs(14)

Servings: 4
Cooking Time: 25 Minutes
Ingredients:
- 1 lb ground beef
- 1 tsp fresh rosemary, chopped
- 1 tbsp garlic, chopped
- 1/2 tsp pepper
- 1 tsp garlic powder
- 1 tsp onion powder
- 1/4 cup breadcrumbs
- 2 eggs
- 1 lb ground pork
- 1/2 tsp pepper
- 1 tsp sea salt

Directions:
1. Fit the oven with the rack in position
2. Add all ingredients into the mixing bowl and mix until well combined.
3. Make small balls from the meat mixture and place it into the parchment-lined baking pan.
4. Set to bake at 400 F for 30 minutes. After 5 minutes place the baking pan in the preheated oven.
5. Serve and enjoy.

Nutrition Info: Calories 441 Fat 13.7 g Carbohydrates 7.2 g Sugar 1 g Protein 68.1 g Cholesterol 266 mg

375.Char Siu

Servings: 4
Cooking Time: 15 Minutes
Ingredients:
- ¼ cup honey
- 1 teaspoon Chinese five-spice powder
- 1 tablespoon Shaoxing wine (rice cooking wine)
- 1 tablespoon hoisin sauce
- 2 teaspoons minced garlic
- 2 teaspoons minced fresh ginger
- 2 tablespoons soy sauce

- 1 tablespoon sugar
- 1 pound (454 g) fatty pork shoulder, cut into long, 1-inch-thick pieces
- Cooking spray

Directions:
1. Combine all the ingredients, except for the pork should, in a microwave-safe bowl. Stir to mix well. Microwave until the honey has dissolved. Stir periodically.
2. Pierce the pork pieces generously with a fork, then put the pork in a large bowl. Pour in half of the honey mixture. Set the remaining sauce aside until ready to serve.
3. Press the pork pieces into the mixture to coat and wrap the bowl in plastic and refrigerate to marinate for at least 8 hours.
4. Spritz the air fryer basket with cooking spray.
5. Discard the marinade and transfer the pork pieces in the basket.
6. Put the air fryer basket on the baking pan and slide into Rack Position 2, select Air Fry, set temperature to 400ºF (205ºC) and set time to 15 minutes.
7. Flip the pork halfway through.
8. When cooking is complete, the pork should be well browned.
9. Meanwhile, microwave the remaining marinade on high for a minute or until it has a thick consistency. Stir periodically.
10. Remove the pork from the oven and allow to cool for 10 minutes before serving with the thickened marinade.

376.Caraway Crusted Beef Steaks

Servings: 4
Cooking Time: 10 Minutes
Ingredients:
- 4 beef steaks
- 2 teaspoons caraway seeds
- 2 teaspoons garlic powder
- Sea salt and cayenne pepper, to taste
- 1 tablespoon melted butter
- $^1/_3$ cup almond flour
- 2 eggs, beaten

Directions:
1. Add the beef steaks to a large bowl and toss with the caraway seeds, garlic powder, salt and pepper until well coated.
2. Stir together the melted butter and almond flour in a bowl. Whisk the eggs in a different bowl.
3. Dredge the seasoned steaks in the eggs, then dip in the almond and butter mixture.
4. Arrange the coated steaks in the basket.
5. Put the air fryer basket on the baking pan and slide into Rack Position 2, select Air Fry, set

temperature to 355ºF (179ºC) and set time to 10 minutes.
6. Flip the steaks once halfway through to ensure even cooking.
7. When cooking is complete, the internal temperature of the beef steaks should reach at least 145ºF (63ºC) on a meat thermometer.
8. Transfer the steaks to plates. Let cool for 5 minutes and serve hot.

377.Chicken Casserole With Coconut

Servings: 4
Cooking Time: 20 Minutes
Ingredients:
- 2 large eggs
- 1 tsp garlic powder
- Salt and black pepper to taste
- ¾ cup breadcrumbs
- ¾ cup shredded coconut
- 1 lb chicken tenders

Directions:
1. Preheat Breville on AirFry function to 400 F. In a wide dish, whisk eggs with garlic powder, pepper, and salt. In another bowl, mix the breadcrumbs and coconut.
2. Dip the chicken tenders in eggs, then in the coconut mix; shake off any excess. Place the prepared chicken tenders in the basket and press Start. Cook for 12-14 minutes until golden.

378.Parmesan Cajun Pork Chops

Servings: 2
Cooking Time: 9 Minutes
Ingredients:
- 2 pork chops, boneless
- 1 tsp dried mixed herbs
- 1 tsp paprika
- 3 tbsp parmesan cheese, grated
- 1 tsp Cajun seasoning
- 1/3 cup almond flour

Directions:
1. Fit the oven with the rack in position 2.
2. Line the air fryer basket with parchment paper.
3. In a shallow dish, mix parmesan cheese, almond flour, paprika, mixed herbs, and Cajun seasoning.
4. Spray pork chops with cooking spray and coat with parmesan cheese.
5. Place coated pork chops in the air fryer basket then place an air fryer basket in the baking pan.
6. Place a baking pan on the oven rack. Set to air fry at 350 F for 9 minutes.
7. Serve and enjoy.

Nutrition Info: Calories 324 Fat 24.8 g
Carbohydrates 2.2 g Sugar 0.3 g Protein 22.9 g
Cholesterol 77 mg

379.Teriyaki Chicken Thighs With Lemony Snow Peas

Servings: 4
Cooking Time: 34 Minutes
Ingredients:
- ¼ cup chicken broth
- ½ teaspoon grated fresh ginger
- ⅛ teaspoon red pepper flakes
- 1½ tablespoons soy sauce
- 4 (5-ounce / 142-g) bone-in chicken thighs, trimmed
- 1 tablespoon mirin
- ½ teaspoon cornstarch
- 1 tablespoon sugar
- 6 ounces (170 g) snow peas, strings removed
- ⅛ teaspoon lemon zest
- 1 garlic clove, minced
- ¼ teaspoon salt
- Ground black pepper, to taste
- ½ teaspoon lemon juice

Directions:
1. Combine the broth, ginger, pepper flakes, and soy sauce in a large bowl. Stir to mix well.
2. Pierce 10 to 15 holes into the chicken skin. Put the chicken in the broth mixture and toss to coat well. Let sit for 10 minutes to marinate.
3. Transfer the marinated chicken on a plate and pat dry with paper towels.
4. Scoop 2 tablespoons of marinade in a microwave-safe bowl and combine with mirin, cornstarch and sugar. Stir to mix well. Microwave for 1 minute or until frothy and has a thick consistency. Set aside.
5. Arrange the chicken in the air fryer basket, skin side up.
6. Put the air fryer basket on the baking pan and slide into Rack Position 2, select Air Fry, set temperature to 400ºF (205ºC) and set time to 25 minutes.
7. Flip the chicken halfway through.
8. When cooking is complete, brush the chicken skin with marinade mixture. Air fry the chicken for 5 more minutes or until glazed.
9. Remove the chicken from the oven. Allow the chicken to cool for 10 minutes.
10. Meanwhile, combine the snow peas, lemon zest, garlic, salt, and ground black pepper in a small bowl. Toss to coat well.
11. Transfer the snow peas in the basket.
12. Put the air fryer basket on the baking pan and slide into Rack Position 2, select Air Fry, set temperature to 400ºF (205ºC) and set time to 3 minutes.
13. When cooking is complete, the peas should be soft.
14. Remove the peas from the oven and toss with lemon juice.
15. Serve the chicken with lemony snow peas.

380.Crunchy Parmesan Pork Chops

Servings: 4
Cooking Time: 10 Minutes
Ingredients:
- 4 pork chops, boneless
- 2 tbsp olive oil
- 1/4 tsp pepper
- 1/2 tsp garlic powder
- 1 tsp dried parsley
- 1/4 tsp smoked paprika
- 2 tbsp breadcrumbs
- 1/4 cup parmesan cheese, grated

Directions:
1. Fit the oven with the rack in position
2. In a shallow dish, mix breadcrumbs, paprika, parmesan cheese, garlic powder, parsley, and pepper.
3. Brush pork chops with oil and coat with breadcrumb mixture.
4. Place coated pork chops into the baking pan.
5. Set to bake at 450 F for 15 minutes. After 5 minutes place the baking pan in the preheated oven.
6. Serve and enjoy.
Nutrition Info: Calories 350 Fat 28.3 g
Carbohydrates 3.1 g Sugar 0.3 g Protein 20.4 g
Cholesterol 73 mg

381.Pork Wonton Wonderful

Servings: 3
Cooking Time: 25 Minutes
Ingredients:
- 8 wanton wrappers (Leasa brand works great, though any will do)
- 4 ounces of raw minced pork
- 1 medium-sized green apple
- 1 cup of water, for wetting the wanton wrappers
- 1 tablespoon of vegetable oil
- ½ tablespoon of oyster sauce
- 1 tablespoon of soy sauce
- Large pinch of ground white pepper

Directions:
1. Preparing the Ingredients. Cover the basket of the air fryer oven with a lining of tin foil, leaving the edges uncovered to allow air to circulate through the basket. Preheat the air fryer oven to 350 degrees.

2.   In a small mixing bowl, combine the oyster sauce, soy sauce, and white pepper, then add in the minced pork and stir thoroughly. Cover and set in the fridge to marinate for at least 15 minutes. Core the apple, and slice into small cubes – smaller than bite-sized chunks.

3.   Add the apples to the marinating meat mixture, and combine thoroughly. Spread the wonton wrappers, and fill each with a large spoonful of the filling. Wrap the wontons into triangles, so that the wrappers fully cover the filling, and seal with a drop of the water.

4.   Coat each filled and wrapped wonton thoroughly with the vegetable oil, to help ensure a nice crispy fry. Place the wontons on the foil-lined air-fryer rack/basket. Place the Rack on the middle-shelf of the air fryer oven.

5.   Air Frying. Set the air fryer oven timer to 25 minutes. Halfway through cooking time, shake the handle of the air fryer rack/basket vigorously to jostle the wontons and ensure even frying. After 25 minutes, when the air fryer oven shuts off, the wontons will be crispy golden-brown on the outside and juicy and delicious on the inside. Serve directly from the Oven rack/basket and enjoy while hot.

382.Chicken With Avocado & Radish Bowl

Servings: 2
Cooking Time: 20 Minutes
Ingredients:
- 2 chicken breasts
- 1 avocado, sliced
- 4 radishes, sliced
- 1 tbsp chopped parsley
- Salt and black pepper to taste

Directions:
1.   Preheat on Air Fry function to 300 F. Cut the chicken into small cubes. Combine all ingredients in a bowl and transfer to the Air Fryer pan. Cook for 14 minutes, shaking once. Serve with cooked rice or fried red kidney beans.

383.Italian Veggie Chicken

Servings: 4
Cooking Time: 30 Minutes
Ingredients:
- 4 chicken breasts
- 1 cup mozzarella cheese, shredded
- 6 bacon slices, cooked & chopped
- 8 oz can artichoke hearts, sliced
- 1 cup cherry tomatoes, cut in half
- 1 zucchini, sliced
- 1 tbsp dried basil

- 1/4 tsp salt

Directions:
1.   Fit the oven with the rack in position
2.   Place chicken breasts into the casserole dish and sprinkle with basil and salt.
3.   Spread artichoke hearts, cherry tomatoes, and zucchini on top of chicken.
4.   Sprinkle shredded cheese and bacon on top of vegetables.
5.   Set to bake at 375 F for 35 minutes. After 5 minutes place the casserole dish in the preheated oven.
6.   Serve and enjoy.

Nutrition Info: Calories 484 Fat 24.2 g Carbohydrates 6.9 g Sugar 2.5 g Protein 56.8 g Cholesterol 165 mg

384.Cheesy Turkey Burgers

Servings: 4
Cooking Time: 25 Minutes
Ingredients:
- 2 medium yellow onions
- 1 tablespoon olive oil
- 1½ teaspoons kosher salt, divided
- 1¼ pound (567 g) ground turkey
- $^1/_3$ cup mayonnaise
- 1 tablespoon Dijon mustard
- 2 teaspoons Worcestershire sauce
- 4 slices sharp Cheddar cheese (about 4 ounces / 113 g in total)
- 4 hamburger buns, sliced

Directions:
1.   Trim the onions and cut them in half through the root. Cut one of the halves in half. Grate one quarter. Place the grated onion in a large bowl. Thinly slice the remaining onions and place in a medium bowl with the oil and ½ teaspoon of kosher salt. Toss to coat. Place the onions in a single layer in the baking pan.
2.   Slide the baking pan into Rack Position 2, select Roast, set temperature to 350ºF (180ºC), and set time to 10 minutes.
3.   While the onions are cooking, add the turkey to the grated onion. Add the remaining kosher salt, mayonnaise, mustard, and Worcestershire sauce. Mix just until combined, being careful not to overwork the turkey. Divide the mixture into 4 patties, each about ¾-inch thick.
4.   When cooking is complete, remove from the oven. Move the onions to one side of the pan and place the burgers on the pan. Poke your finger into the center of each burger to make a deep indentation.
5.   Select Convection Broil, set temperature to High, and set time to 12 minutes.

6. After 6 minutes, remove the pan. Turn the burgers and stir the onions. Return the pan to the oven and continue cooking. After about 4 minutes, remove the pan and place the cheese slices on the burgers. Return the pan to the oven and continue cooking for about 1 minute, or until the cheese is melted and the center of the burgers has reached at least 165ºF (74ºC) on a meat thermometer.
7. When cooking is complete, remove from the oven. Loosely cover the burgers with foil.
8. Lay out the buns, cut-side up, on the oven rack. Select Convection Broil; set temperature to High, and set time to 3 minutes. Check the buns after 2 minutes; they should be lightly browned.
9. Remove the buns from the oven. Assemble the burgers and serve.

385.Cheesy Chicken With Tomato Sauce

Servings: 2
Cooking Time: 20 Minutes
Ingredients:
- 2 chicken breasts, ½-inch thick
- 1 egg, beaten
- ½ cup breadcrumbs
- Salt and black pepper to taste
- 2 tbsp tomato sauce
- 2 tbsp Grana Padano cheese, grated
- ¼ cup mozzarella cheese, shredded

Directions:
1. Preheat Breville on AirFry function to 350 F. Dip the breasts into the egg, then into the crumbs and arrange on the greased basket. Cook for 5 minutes. Turn, drizzle with tomato sauce, sprinkle with Grana Padano and mozzarella cheeses, and cook for 5 more minutes. Serve warm.

386.Flavors Cheesy Chicken Breasts

Servings: 6
Cooking Time: 45 Minutes
Ingredients:
- 3 lbs chicken breasts, sliced in half
- 1 tsp garlic powder
- 1/2 cup parmesan cheese, shredded
- 1 cup Greek yogurt
- 1/2 tsp pepper
- 1/2 tsp salt

Directions:
1. Fit the oven with the rack in position
2. Place chicken breasts into the greased baking dish.
3. Mix parmesan cheese, yogurt, garlic powder, pepper, and salt and pour over chicken.

4. Set to bake at 375 F for 50 minutes. After 5 minutes place the baking dish in the preheated oven.
5. Serve and enjoy.
Nutrition Info: Calories 482 Fat 19.1 g Carbohydrates 2.1 g Sugar 1.5 g Protein 71.5 g Cholesterol 209 mg

387.Enchilada Cheese Chicken

Servings: 3
Cooking Time: 25 Minutes
Ingredients:
- 3 cups chicken breasts, chopped
- 2 cups cheese, grated
- ½ cup salsa
- 1 can green chilies, chopped
- 12 flour tortillas
- 2 cans enchilada sauce

Directions:
1. In a bowl, mix salsa and enchilada sauce. Toss in the chopped chicken to coat. Place the chicken on the tortillas and roll; top with cheese. Place the prepared tortillas in a baking tray and cook for 15-18 minutes at 400 F on Bake function. Serve with guacamole and hot dips!

388.Drumsticks With Barbecue-honey Sauce

Servings: 5
Cooking Time: 18 Minutes
Ingredients:
- 1 tablespoon olive oil
- 10 chicken drumsticks
- Chicken seasoning or rub, to taste
- Salt and ground black pepper, to taste
- 1 cup barbecue sauce
- ¼ cup honey

Directions:
1. Grease the basket with olive oil.
2. Rub the chicken drumsticks with chicken seasoning or rub, salt and ground black pepper on a clean work surface.
3. Arrange the chicken drumsticks in the basket.
4. Put the air fryer basket on the baking pan and slide into Rack Position 2, select Air Fry, set temperature to 390ºF (199ºC) and set time to 18 minutes.
5. Flip the drumsticks halfway through.
6. When cooking is complete, the drumsticks should be lightly browned.
7. Meanwhile, combine the barbecue sauce and honey in a small bowl. Stir to mix well.
8. Remove the drumsticks from the oven and baste with the sauce mixture to serve.

389.Ravioli With Beef-marinara Sauce

Servings: 4
Cooking Time: 10 Minutes
Ingredients:
- 1 (20-ounce / 567-g) package frozen cheese ravioli
- 1 teaspoon kosher salt
- 1¼ cups water
- 6 ounces (170 g) cooked ground beef
- 2½ cups Marinara sauce
- ¼ cup grated Parmesan cheese, for garnish

Directions:
1. Place the ravioli in an even layer in the baking pan. Stir the salt into the water until dissolved and pour it over the ravioli.
2. Slide the baking pan into Rack Position 1, select Convection Bake, set temperature to 450ºF (235ºC), and set time to 10 minutes.
3. While the ravioli is cooking, mix the ground beef into the marinara sauce in a medium bowl.
4. After 6 minutes, remove the pan from the oven. Blot off any remaining water, or drain the ravioli and return them to the pan. Pour the meat sauce over the ravioli. Return the pan to the oven and continue cooking.
5. When cooking is complete, the ravioli should be tender and sauce heated through. Gently stir the ingredients. Serve the ravioli with the Parmesan cheese, if desired.

390.Mom's Meatballs

Servings: 4
Cooking Time: 20 Minutes
Ingredients:
- 1 lb ground beef
- 2 tbsp olive oil
- 1 red onion, chopped
- 1 garlic clove, minced
- 2 whole eggs, beaten
- Salt and black pepper to taste

Directions:
1. Warm olive oil in a pan over medium heat and sauté onion and garlic for 3 minutes until tender; transfer to a bowl. Add in ground beef and egg and mix well. Season with salt and pepper.
2. Preheat Breville oven to 360 F on AirFry function. Mold the mixture into golf-size ball shapes. Place the balls in the greased frying basket and cook for 12-14 minutes. Serve.

391.Thai Game Hens With Cucumber And Chile Salad

Servings: 6
Cooking Time: 25 Minutes
Ingredients:
- 2 (1¼-pound / 567-g) Cornish game hens, giblets discarded
- 1 tablespoon fish sauce
- 6 tablespoons chopped fresh cilantro
- 2 teaspoons lime zest
- 1 teaspoon ground coriander
- 2 garlic cloves, minced
- 2 tablespoons packed light brown sugar
- 2 teaspoons vegetable oil
- Salt and ground black pepper, to taste
- 1 English cucumber, halved lengthwise and sliced thin
- 1 Thai chile, stemmed, deseeded, and minced
- 2 tablespoons chopped dry-roasted peanuts
- 1 small shallot, sliced thinly
- 1 tablespoon lime juice
- Lime wedges, for serving
- Cooking spray

Directions:
1. Arrange a game hen on a clean work surface, remove the backbone with kitchen shears, then pound the hen breast to flat. Cut the breast in half. Repeat with the remaining game hen.
2. Loose the breast and thigh skin with your fingers, then pat the game hens dry and pierce about 10 holes into the fat deposits of the hens. Tuck the wings under the hens.
3. Combine 2 teaspoons of fish sauce, ¼ cup of cilantro, lime zest, coriander, garlic, 4 teaspoons of sugar, 1 teaspoon of vegetable oil, ½ teaspoon of salt, and ⅛ teaspoon of ground black pepper in a small bowl. Stir to mix well.
4. Rub the fish sauce mixture under the breast and thigh skin of the game hens, then let sit for 10 minutes to marinate.
5. Spritz the air fryer basket with cooking spray.
6. Arrange the marinated game hens in the basket, skin side down.
7. Put the air fryer basket on the baking pan and slide into Rack Position 2, select Air Fry, set temperature to 400ºF (205ºC) and set time to 25 minutes.
8. Flip the game hens halfway through the cooking time.
9. When cooking is complete, the hen skin should be golden brown and the internal temperature of the hens should read at least 165ºF (74ºC).
10. Meanwhile, combine all the remaining ingredients, except for the lime wedges, in a large bowl and sprinkle with salt and black pepper. Toss to mix well.

11. Transfer the fried hens on a large plate, then sit the salad aside and squeeze the lime wedges over before serving.

392.Air Fry Chicken Drumsticks

Servings: 6
Cooking Time: 25 Minutes
Ingredients:
- 6 chicken drumsticks
- 1/2 tsp garlic powder
- 2 tbsp olive oil
- 1/2 tsp ground cumin
- 3/4 tsp paprika
- Pepper
- Salt

Directions:
1. Fit the oven with the rack in position 2.
2. Add chicken drumsticks and olive oil in a large bowl and toss well.
3. Sprinkle garlic powder, paprika, cumin, pepper, and salt over chicken drumsticks and toss until well coated.
4. Place chicken drumsticks in the air fryer basket then place an air fryer basket in the baking pan.
5. Place a baking pan on the oven rack. Set to air fry at 400 F for 25 minutes.
6. Serve and enjoy.
Nutrition Info: Calories 120 Fat 7.4 g Carbohydrates 0.4 g Sugar 0.1 g Protein 12.8 g Cholesterol 40 mg

393.Cheesy Bacon Chicken

Servings: 4
Cooking Time: 30 Minutes
Ingredients:
- 4 chicken breasts, sliced in half
- 1 cup cheddar cheese, shredded
- 8 bacon slices, cooked & chopped
- 6 oz cream cheese
- Pepper
- Salt

Directions:
1. Fit the oven with the rack in position
2. Place season chicken with pepper and salt and place it into the greased baking dish.
3. Add cream cheese and bacon on top of chicken.
4. Sprinkle shredded cheddar cheese on top of chicken.
5. Set to bake at 400 F for 35 minutes. After 5 minutes place the baking dish in the preheated oven.
6. Serve and enjoy.
Nutrition Info: Calories 745 Fat 50.9 g Carbohydrates 2.1 g Sugar 0.2 g Protein 66.6 g Cholesterol 248 mg

394.Easy Pork Bites

Servings: 4
Cooking Time: 15 Minutes
Ingredients:
- 1 lb pork belly, cut into 3/4-inch cubes
- 1/2 tsp onion powder
- 1/2 tsp garlic powder
- 1 tsp soy sauce
- Pepper
- Salt

Directions:
1. Fit the oven with the rack in position 2.
2. In a mixing bowl, toss pork cubes with onion powder, garlic powder, soy sauce, pepper, and salt.
3. Place pork cubes in the air fryer basket then place an air fryer basket in the baking pan.
4. Place a baking pan on the oven rack. Set to air fry at 400 F for 15 minutes.
5. Serve and enjoy.
Nutrition Info: Calories 526 Fat 30.5 g Carbohydrates 0.6 g Sugar 0.2 g Protein 52.5 g Cholesterol 131 mg

395.Reuben Beef Rolls With Thousand Island Sauce

Servings: 10 Rolls
Cooking Time: 10 Minutes
Ingredients:
- ½ pound (227 g) cooked corned beef, chopped
- ½ cup drained and chopped sauerkraut
- 1 (8-ounce / 227-g) package cream cheese, softened
- ½ cup shredded Swiss cheese
- 20 slices prosciutto
- Cooking spray
- Thousand Island Sauce:
- ¼ cup chopped dill pickles
- ¼ cup tomato sauce
- ¾ cup mayonnaise
- Fresh thyme leaves, for garnish
- 2 tablespoons sugar
- ⅛ teaspoon fine sea salt
- Ground black pepper, to taste

Directions:
1. Spritz the air fryer basket with cooking spray.
2. Combine the beef, sauerkraut, cream cheese, and Swiss cheese in a large bowl. Stir to mix well.
3. Unroll a slice of prosciutto on a clean work surface, then top with another slice of prosciutto crosswise. Scoop up 4 tablespoons of the beef mixture in the center.

4. Fold the top slice sides over the filling as the ends of the roll, then roll up the long sides of the bottom prosciutto and make it into a roll shape. Overlap the sides by about 1 inch. Repeat with remaining filling and prosciutto.
5. Arrange the rolls in the prepared pan, seam side down, and spritz with cooking spray.
6. Put the air fryer basket on the baking pan and slide into Rack Position 2, select Air Fry, set temperature to 400ºF (205ºC) and set time to 10 minutes.
7. Flip the rolls halfway through.
8. When cooking is complete, the rolls should be golden and crispy.
9. Meanwhile, combine the ingredients for the sauce in a small bowl. Stir to mix well.
10. Serve the rolls with the dipping sauce.

396.Chicken Fried Baked Pastry

Ingredients:
- 1 or 2 green chilies that are finely chopped or mashed
- ½ tsp. cumin
- 1 tsp. coarsely crushed coriander
- 1 dry red chili broken into pieces
- A small amount of salt (to taste)
- 2 tbsp. unsalted butter
- 1 ½ cup all-purpose flour
- A pinch of salt to taste
- Add as much water as required to make the dough stiff and firm
- 1 lb. chicken (Remove the chicken from the bone and cut it into pieces)
- ¼ cup boiled peas
- 1 tsp. powdered ginger
- ½ tsp. dried mango powder
- ½ tsp. red chili power.
- 1-2 tbsp. coriander.

Directions:
1. You will first need to make the outer covering. In a large bowl, add the flour, butter and enough water to knead it into dough that is stiff. Transfer this to a container and leave it to rest for five minutes.
2. Place a pan on medium flame and add the oil. Roast the mustard seeds and once roasted, add the coriander seeds and the chopped dry red chilies. Add all the dry ingredients for the filling and mix the ingredients well.
3. Add a little water and continue to stir the ingredients. Make small balls out of the dough and roll them out. Cut the rolled-out dough into halves and apply a little water on the edges to help you fold the halves into a cone. Add the filling to the cone and close up the samosa. Pre-heat the oven for around 5 to 6 minutes at 300 Fahrenheit.

4. Place all the samosas in the fry basket and close the basket properly. Keep the oven at 200 degrees for another 20 to 25 minutes. Around the halfway point, open the basket and turn the samosas over for uniform cooking.
5. After this, fry at 250 degrees for around 10 minutes in order to give them the desired golden-brown color. Serve hot. Recommended sides are tamarind or mint sauce.

397.Crunchy Chicken Tenderloins

Servings: 4
Cooking Time: 20 Minutes
Ingredients:
- 8 chicken tenderloins
- 2 tbsp butter, melted
- 2 oz breadcrumbs
- 1 large egg, whisked

Directions:
1. Preheat Breville on AirFry function to 380 F. Dip the chicken in the egg. Then roll up them the crumbs. Drizzle with melted butter and arrange on the frying basket. Press Start and cook for 12-14 minutes. Set to Broil function for crispier taste. Serve warm.

398.Mustard Chicken Thighs

Servings: 4
Cooking Time: 50 Minutes
Ingredients:
- 1 1/2 lbs chicken thighs, skinless and boneless
- 2 tbsp Dijon mustard
- 1/4 cup French mustard
- 1/4 cup maple syrup
- 1 tbsp olive oil

Directions:
1. Fit the oven with the rack in position
2. In a bowl, mix maple syrup, olive oil, Dijon mustard, and French mustard.
3. Add chicken to the bowl and coat well.
4. Arrange chicken in a baking dish.
5. Set to bake at 375 F for 55 minutes. After 5 minutes place the baking dish in the preheated oven.
6. Serve and enjoy.
Nutrition Info: Calories 410 Fat 16.5 g Carbohydrates 13.6 g Sugar 11.8 g Protein 49.6 g Cholesterol 151 mg

399.Juicy Baked Chicken Breast

Servings: 4
Cooking Time: 25 Minutes
Ingredients:
- 4 chicken breasts

- 1 tbsp fresh parsley, chopped
- 1/4 tsp red pepper flakes
- 1/2 tsp black pepper
- 1 tsp Italian seasoning
- 2 tbsp olive oil
- 1/4 cup balsamic vinegar
- 1 tsp kosher salt

Directions:
1. Fit the oven with the rack in position
2. Place chicken breasts into the mixing bowl.
3. Mix together remaining ingredients and pour over chicken breasts and coat well and let marinate for 30 minutes.
4. Arrange marinated chicken breasts into a greased baking dish.
5. Set to bake at 425 F for 30 minutes. After 5 minutes place the baking dish in the preheated oven.
6. Slice and serve.

Nutrition Info: Calories 345 Fat 18.2 g Carbohydrates 0.6 g Sugar 0.2 g Protein 42.3 g Cholesterol 131 mg

SNACKS AND DESSERTS RECIPES

400.Blackberry Crisp

Servings: 4
Cooking Time: 30 Minutes
Ingredients:
- 1 cup Crunchy Granola
- 2 cups blackberries
- ⅓ cup powdered erythritol
- 2 tbsp. lemon juice
- ¼ tsp. xanthan gum

Directions:
1. Take a large bowl, toss blackberries, erythritol, lemon juice and xanthan gum.
2. Pour into 6-inch round baking dish and cover with foil. Place into the air fryer basket.
3. Adjust the temperature to 350 Degrees F and set the timer for 12 minutes.
4. When the timer beeps, remove the foil and stir.
5. Sprinkle granola over mixture and return to the air fryer basket. Adjust the temperature to 320 Degrees F and set the timer for 3 minutes or until top is golden. Serve warm.
Nutrition Info: Calories: 496; Protein: 9.2g; Fiber: 12.5g; Fat: 42.1g; Carbs: 44.0g

401.Blueberry Cakes

Ingredients:
- 1 cup sugar
- 3 tsp. vinegar
- 2 cups blueberries
- ½ tsp. vanilla essence
- 2 cups All-purpose flour
- 1 ½ cup milk
- ½ tsp. baking powder
- ½ tsp. baking soda
- 2 tbsp. butter
- Muffin cups or butter paper cups.

Directions:
1. Mix the ingredients together and use your Oregano Fingers to get a crumbly mixture.
2. Add the baking soda and the vinegar to the milk and mix continuously. Add this milk to the mixture and create a batter that you will need to transfer to the muffin cups.
3. Preheat the fryer to 300 Fahrenheit for five minutes. You will need to place the muffin cups in the basket and cover it. Cook the muffins for fifteen minutes and check whether or not the muffins are cooked using a toothpick.
4. Remove the cups and serve hot.

402.Spiced Avocado Pudding

Servings: 6
Cooking Time: 15 Minutes
Ingredients:
- 4 small avocados, peeled, pitted and mashed
- 2 eggs, whisked
- ¾ cup swerve
- 1 cup coconut milk
- 1 tsp. cinnamon powder
- ½ tsp. ginger powder

Directions:
1. Take a bowl and mix all the ingredients and whisk well.
2. Pour into a pudding mould, put it in the air fryer and cook at 350°F for 25 minutes. Serve warm
Nutrition Info: Calories: 192; Fat: 8g; Fiber: 2g; Carbs: 5g; Protein: 4g

403.Air Fried Chicken Wings

Servings: 4
Cooking Time: 18 Minutes
Ingredients:
- 2 pounds (907 g) chicken wings
- Cooking spray

Directions:
1. Marinade:
2. cup buttermilk
3. ½ teaspoon salt
4. ½ teaspoon black pepper
5. Coating:
6. cup flour
7. cup panko bread crumbs
8. tablespoons poultry seasoning
9. teaspoons salt
10. Whisk together all the ingredients for the marinade in a large bowl.
11. Add the chicken wings to the marinade and toss well. Transfer to the refrigerator to marinate for at least an hour.
12. Spritz the air fryer basket with cooking spray. Set aside.
13. Thoroughly combine all the ingredients for the coating in a shallow bowl.
14. Remove the chicken wings from the marinade and shake off any excess. Roll them in the coating mixture.
15. Place the chicken wings in the basket in a single layer. Mist the wings with cooking spray.
16. Put the air fryer basket on the baking pan and slide into Rack Position 2, select Air Fry, set temperature to 360°F (182°C), and set time to 18 minutes.

17. Flip the wings halfway through the cooking time.
18. When cooking is complete, the wings should be crisp and golden brown on the outside. Remove from the oven to a plate and serve hot.

minutes, or until the custard is set. Remove from the oven and sprinkle lightly with cinnamon.
6. Serve warm.

404.Air Fryer Cinnamon Rolls

Servings: 8
Cooking Time: 5 Minutes
Ingredients:
- 1 ½ tbsp. cinnamon
- ¾ C. brown sugar
- ¼ C. melted coconut oil
- 1 pound frozen bread dough, thawed
- Glaze:
- ½ tsp. vanilla
- 1 ¼ C. powdered erythritol
- 2 tbsp. softened ghee
- 3 ounces softened cream cheese

Directions:
1. Preparing the Ingredients. Lay out bread dough and roll out into a rectangle. Brush melted ghee over dough and leave a 1-inch border along edges.
2. Mix cinnamon and sweetener together and then sprinkle over the dough.
3. Roll dough tightly and slice into 8 pieces. Let sit 1-2 hours to rise.
4. To make the glaze, simply mix ingredients together till smooth.
5. Air Frying. Once rolls rise, place into the air fryer oven and cook 5 minutes at 350 degrees.
6. Serve rolls drizzled in cream cheese glaze. Enjoy!
Nutrition Info: CALORIES: 390; FAT:8G; PROTEIN:1G; SUGAR:7G

405.Cinnamon Rice Pudding

Ingredients:
- 5 large eggs, beaten
- 2 cups heavy cream
- 1 tsp vanilla extract
- Sprinkle of ground cinnamon, for garnish
- 1 Tbsp butter
- 2 cups cooked white rice
- ½ tsp ground cinnamon
- ¾ cup sugar

Directions:
1. Preheat the oven to 350°F.
2. Butter the inside of a 2-quart oven and put the rice in the pot.
3. In a large bowl, mix the cinnamon, sugar, and eggs until well blended.
4. Whisk in the cream and vanilla.
5. Pour the mixture gently over the rice. Cover with the lid and place oven in the oven. Bake for 50

406.Vanilla Lemon Cupcakes

Servings: 6
Cooking Time: 15 Minutes
Ingredients:
- 1 egg
- 1/2 cup milk
- 2 tbsp canola oil
- 1/4 tsp baking soda
- 3/4 tsp baking powder
- 1 tsp lemon zest, grated
- 1/2 cup sugar
- 1 cup flour
- 1/2 tsp vanilla
- 1/2 tsp salt

Directions:
1. Fit the oven with the rack in position
2. Line 12-cups muffin tin with cupcake liners and set aside.
3. In a bowl, whisk egg, vanilla, milk, oil, and sugar until creamy.
4. Add remaining ingredients and stir until just combined.
5. Pour batter into the prepared muffin tin.
6. Set to bake at 350 F for 20 minutes. After 5 minutes place muffin tin in the preheated oven.
7. Serve and enjoy.
Nutrition Info: Calories 200 Fat 6 g Carbohydrates 35 g Sugar 17 g Protein 3 g Cholesterol 30 mg

407.Orange Coconut Cake

Servings: 6
Cooking Time: 17 Minutes
Ingredients:
- 1 stick butter, melted
- ¾ cup granulated Swerve
- 2 eggs, beaten
- ¾ cup coconut flour
- ¼ teaspoon salt
- $1/3$ teaspoon grated nutmeg
- $1/3$ cup coconut milk
- 1¼ cups almond flour
- ½ teaspoon baking powder
- 2 tablespoons unsweetened orange jam
- Cooking spray

Directions:
1. Coat the baking pan with cooking spray. Set aside.
2. In a large mixing bowl, whisk together the melted butter and granulated Swerve until fluffy.

3. Mix in the beaten eggs and whisk again until smooth. Stir in the coconut flour, salt, and nutmeg and gradually pour in the coconut milk. Add the remaining ingredients and stir until well incorporated.
4. Scrape the batter into the baking pan.
5. Slide the baking pan into Rack Position 1, select Convection Bake, set temperature to 355ºF (179ºC), and set time to 17 minutes.
6. When cooking is complete, the top of the cake should spring back when gently pressed with your fingers.
7. Remove from the oven to a wire rack to cool. Serve chilled.

408.Healthy Carrot Fries

Servings: 4
Cooking Time: 25 Minutes
Ingredients:
- 4 medium carrots, peel and cut into fries shape
- 1/2 tbsp paprika
- 1 1/2 tbsp olive oil
- 1/2 tsp salt

Directions:
1. Fit the oven with the rack in position
2. Add carrots, paprika, oil, and salt into the mixing bowl and toss well.
3. Transfer carrot fries in baking pan.
4. Set to bake at 450 F for 30 minutes. After 5 minutes place the baking pan in the preheated oven.
5. Serve and enjoy.
Nutrition Info: Calories 73 Fat 5.4 g Carbohydrates 6.5 g Sugar 3.1 g Protein 0.6 g Cholesterol 0 mg

409.Tasty Broccoli Fritters

Servings: 4
Cooking Time: 30 Minutes
Ingredients:
- 3 cups broccoli florets, steam & chopped
- 2 eggs, lightly beaten
- 2 garlic cloves, minced
- 2 cups cheddar cheese, shredded
- 1/4 cup breadcrumbs
- 1/2 tsp Italian seasoning
- Pepper
- Salt

Directions:
1. Fit the oven with the rack in position
2. Add all ingredients into the large bowl and mix until well combined.
3. Make patties from broccoli mixture and place in baking pan.

4. Set to bake at 375 F for 35 minutes. After 5 minutes place the baking pan in the preheated oven.
5. Serve and enjoy.
Nutrition Info: Calories 313 Fat 21.7 g Carbohydrates 10.9 g Sugar 2.1 g Protein 19.8 g Cholesterol 142 mg

410.Banana Pancakes

Ingredients:
- 4 ripe bananas (shredded)
- Salt and Pepper to taste
- 3 tbsp. Butter
- 1 ½ cups almond flour
- 3 eggs
- 2 tsp. dried basil
- 2 tsp. dried parsley

Directions:
1. Preheat the air fryer to 250 Fahrenheit. In a small bowl, mix the ingredients together. Ensure that the mixture is smooth and well balanced.
2. Take a pancake mold and grease it with butter. Add the batter to the mold and place it in the air fryer basket.
3. Cook till both the sides of the pancake have browned on both sides and serve with maple syrup.

411.Coconut Butter Apple Bars

Servings: 8
Cooking Time: 45 Minutes
Ingredients:
- 1 tbsp ground flax seed
- 1/4 cup coconut butter, softened
- 1 cup pecans
- 1 cup of water
- 1/4 cup dried apples
- 1 1/2 tsp baking powder
- 1 1/2 tsp cinnamon
- 1 tsp vanilla
- 2 tbsp swerve

Directions:
1. Fit the oven with the rack in position
2. Add all ingredients into the blender and blend until smooth.
3. Pour blended mixture into the greased baking dish.
4. Set to bake at 350 F for 50 minutes. After 5 minutes place the baking dish in the preheated oven.
5. Slice and serve.
Nutrition Info: Calories 161 Fat 15 g Carbohydrates 6 g Sugar 2 g Protein 2 g Cholesterol 0 mg

412.Nan Khatam

Ingredients:
- 1 tbsp. Unsalted Butter
- 1 tsp. baking powder
- 1 tsp. baking soda
- 1 tsp. cardamom powder
- 1 ½ cup all-purpose flour
- 1 cup Gram flour
- 1 cup +3 tbsp. icing sugar

Directions:
1. Create a crumbly mixture using the ingredients and make small balls of the mixture and flattening them on a prepared baking tray.
2. Preheat the fryer to 300 Fahrenheit for five minutes. Place the baking tray in the basket and reduce the temperature to 250 Fahrenheit. Cook both sides of the ball for five minutes to ensure that they are cooked uniformly. Once the nan khatam has cooled, store them in an airtight container.

413.Flavorful Crab Dip

Servings: 6
Cooking Time: 15 Minutes
Ingredients:
- 6 oz crab lump meat
- 1 tbsp mayonnaise
- 1/8 tsp paprika
- 1/4 cup sour cream
- 4 tsp bell pepper, diced
- 1 tbsp butter, softened
- 1 tsp parsley, chopped
- 1 tbsp green onion, sliced
- 1/4 cup mozzarella cheese, shredded
- 4 tsp onion, chopped
- 2 oz cream cheese, softened
- 1/4 tsp salt

Directions:
1. Fit the oven with the rack in position
2. In a bowl, mix together cream cheese, butter, sour cream, and mayonnaise until smooth.
3. Add remaining ingredients and stir well.
4. Pour mixture into the greased baking dish.
5. Set to bake at 350 F for 20 minutes. After 5 minutes place the baking dish in the preheated oven.
6. Serve and enjoy.

Nutrition Info: Calories 131 Fat 10.8 g Carbohydrates 8.1 g Sugar 4.3 g Protein 6.4 g Cholesterol 37 mg

414.Chocolate Soufflé

Servings: 2
Cooking Time: 16 Minutes
Ingredients:
- 3 oz. semi-sweet chocolate, chopped
- ¼ cup butter
- 2 eggs, yolks and whites separated
- 3 tablespoons sugar
- ½ teaspoon pure vanilla extract
- 2 tablespoons all-purpose flour
- 1 teaspoon powdered sugar plus extra for dusting

Directions:
1. In a microwave-safe bowl, place the butter, and chocolate. Microwave on high heat for about 2 minutes or until melted completely, stirring after every 30 seconds.
2. Remove from microwave and stir the mixture until smooth.
3. In another bowl, add the egg yolks and whisk well.
4. Add the sugar, and vanilla extract and whisk well.
5. Add the chocolate mixture and mix until well combined.
6. Add the flour and mix well.
7. In a clean glass bowl, add the egg whites and whisk until soft peaks form.
8. Fold the whipped egg whites in 3 portions into the chocolate mixture.
9. Grease 2 ramekins and sprinkle each with a pinch of sugar.
10. Place mixture into the prepared ramekins and with the back of a spoon, smooth the top surface.
11. Press "Power Button" of Air Fry Oven and turn the dial to select the "Air Fry" mode.
12. Press the Time button and again turn the dial to set the cooking time to 14 minutes.
13. Now push the Temp button and rotate the dial to set the temperature at 330 degrees F.
14. Press "Start/Pause" button to start.
15. When the unit beeps to show that it is preheated, open the lid.
16. Arrange the ramekins in "Air Fry Basket" and insert in the oven.
17. Place the ramekins onto a wire rack to cool slightly.
18. Sprinkle with the powdered sugar and serve warm.

Nutrition Info: Calories 591 Total Fat 38.7 g Saturated Fat 23 g Cholesterol 225 mg Sodium 225 mg Total Carbs 52.6 g Fiber 0.2 g Sugar 41.1 g Protein 9.4 g

415.Spicy Cauliflower Florets

Servings: 4
Cooking Time: 15 Minutes
Ingredients:
- 1 medium cauliflower head, cut into florets

- 1/2 tsp old bay seasoning
- 1/4 tsp paprika
- 1/4 tsp cayenne
- 1/4 tsp chili powder
- 1 tbsp garlic, minced
- 3 tbsp olive oil
- Pepper
- Salt

Directions:
1. Fit the oven with the rack in position 2.
2. In a bowl, toss cauliflower with remaining ingredients.
3. Add cauliflower florets in air fryer basket then place air fryer basket in baking pan.
4. Place a baking pan on the oven rack. Set to air fry at 400 F for 15 minutes.
5. Serve and enjoy.

Nutrition Info: Calories 130 Fat 10.7 g Carbohydrates 8.6 g Sugar 3.5 g Protein 3 g Cholesterol 0 mg

416.Fried Bananas With Chocolate Sauce

Servings: 2
Cooking Time: 10 Minutes
Ingredients:
- 1 large egg
- ¼ cup cornstarch
- ¼ cup plain bread crumbs
- 3 bananas, halved crosswise
- Cooking oil
- Chocolate sauce (see Ingredient tip)

Directions:
1. Preparing the Ingredients. In a small bowl, beat the egg. In another bowl, place the cornstarch. Place the bread crumbs in a third bowl. Dip the bananas in the cornstarch, then the egg, and then the bread crumbs.
2. Spray the air fryer rack/basket with cooking oil. Place the bananas in the basket and spray them with cooking oil.
3. Air Frying. Cook for 5 minutes. Open the air fryer oven and flip the bananas. Cook for an additional 2 minutes. Transfer the bananas to plates.
4. Drizzle the chocolate sauce over the bananas, and serve.
5. You can make your own chocolate sauce using 2 tablespoons milk and ¼ cup chocolate chips. Heat a saucepan over medium-high heat. Add the milk and stir for 1 to 2 minutes. Add the chocolate chips. Stir for 2 minutes, or until the chocolate has melted.

Nutrition Info: CALORIES: 203; FAT:6G; PROTEIN:3G; FIBER:3G

417.Honey And Orange Pancakes

Ingredients:
- 2 tsp. dried basil
- 2 tsp. dried parsley
- Salt and Pepper to taste
- 3 tbsp. Butter
- 1 orange (zested)
- 1 ½ cups almond flour
- 3 eggs
- 1 tbsp. honey

Directions:
1. Preheat the air fryer to 250 Fahrenheit.
2. In a small bowl, mix the ingredients together. Ensure that the mixture is smooth and well balanced.
3. Take a pancake mold and grease it with butter. Add the batter to the mold and place it in the air fryer basket.
4. Cook till both the sides of the pancake have browned on both sides and serve with maple syrup.

418.Lemon-raspberry Muffins

Servings: 6
Cooking Time: 15 Minutes
Ingredients:
- 2 cups almond flour
- ¾ cup Swerve
- 1¼ teaspoons baking powder
- $^1/_3$ teaspoon ground allspice
- $^1/_3$ teaspoon ground anise star
- ½ teaspoon grated lemon zest
- ¼ teaspoon salt
- 2 eggs
- 1 cup sour cream
- ½ cup coconut oil
- ½ cup raspberries

Directions:
1. Line a muffin pan with 6 paper liners.
2. In a mixing bowl, mix the almond flour, Swerve, baking powder, allspice, anise, lemon zest, and salt.
3. In another mixing bowl, beat the eggs, sour cream, and coconut oil until well mixed. Add the egg mixture to the flour mixture and stir to combine. Mix in the raspberries.
4. Scrape the batter into the prepared muffin cups, filling each about three-quarters full.
5. Put the muffin pan into Rack Position 1, select Convection Bake, set temperature to 345ºF (174ºC), and set time to 15 minutes.
6. When cooking is complete, the tops should be golden and a toothpick inserted in the middle should come out clean.
7. Allow the muffins to cool for 10 minutes in the muffin pan before removing and serving.

419.Mushroom Platter

Servings: 4
Cooking Time: 15 Minutes
Ingredients:
- 12 oz. Portobello mushrooms; sliced
- 2 tbsp. olive oil
- 2 tbsp. balsamic vinegar
- ½ tsp. rosemary; dried
- ½ tsp. thyme; dried
- ½ tsp. basil; dried
- ½ tsp. tarragon; dried
- A pinch of salt and black pepper

Directions:
1. Take a bowl and mix all the ingredients and toss well.
2. Arrange the mushroom slices in your air fryer's basket and cook at 380°F for 12 minutes. Arrange the mushroom slices on a platter and serve
Nutrition Info: Calories: 147; Fat: 8g; Fiber: 2g; Carbs: 3g; Protein: 3g

420.Easy Blueberry Muffins

Servings: 12
Cooking Time: 30 Minutes
Ingredients:
- 5.5 oz plain yogurt
- ½ cup fresh blueberries
- 2 tsp baking powder, gluten-free
- ¼ cup Swerve
- 2 ½ cups almond flour
- ½ tsp vanilla
- 3 eggs
- Pinch of salt

Directions:
1. Fit the oven with the rack in position
2. Line 6-cups muffin tin with cupcake liners and set aside.
3. In a bowl, whisk egg, yogurt, vanilla, and salt until smooth.
4. Add flour, swerve and baking powder and blend again until smooth.
5. Add blueberries and stir well.
6. Pour batter into the prepared muffin tin.
7. Set to bake at 325 F for 35 minutes. After 5 minutes place muffin tin in the preheated oven.
8. Serve and enjoy.
Nutrition Info: Calories 63 Fat 4.2 g Carbohydrates 3.6 g Sugar 1.8 g Protein 3.4 g Cholesterol 42 mg

421.Bbq Pulled Mushrooms

Servings: 2
Cooking Time: 15 Minutes
Ingredients:
- 4 large portobello mushrooms
- ½ cup low-carb, sugar-free barbecue sauce
- 1 tbsp. salted butter; melted.
- 1 tsp. paprika
- ¼ tsp. onion powder.
- ¼ tsp. ground black pepper
- 1 tsp. chili powder

Directions:
1. Remove stem and scoop out the underside of each mushroom. Brush the caps with butter and sprinkle with pepper, chili powder, paprika and onion powder.
2. Place mushrooms into the air fryer basket. Adjust the temperature to 400 Degrees F and set the timer for 8 minutes.
3. When the timer beeps, remove mushrooms from the basket and place on a cutting board or work surface. Using two forks, gently pull the mushrooms apart, creating strands.
4. Place mushroom strands into a 4-cup round baking dish with barbecue sauce. Place dish into the air fryer basket.
5. Adjust the temperature to 350 Degrees F and set the timer for 4 minutes. Stir halfway through the cooking time. Serve warm.
Nutrition Info: Calories: 108; Protein: 3.3g; Fiber: 2.7g; Fat: 5.9g; Carbs: 10.9g

422.Tasty Potato Wedges

Servings: 4
Cooking Time: 15 Minutes
Ingredients:
- 2 medium potatoes, cut into wedges
- 1/4 tsp garlic powder
- 1/4 tsp pepper
- 1/2 tsp paprika
- 1 1/2 tbsp olive oil
- 1/8 tsp cayenne
- 1 tsp sea salt

Directions:
1. Fit the oven with the rack in position 2.
2. Soak potato wedges into the water for 30 minutes.
3. Drain well and pat dry with a paper towel.
4. In a bowl, toss potato wedges with remaining ingredients.
5. Place potato wedges in the air fryer basket then place an air fryer basket in the baking pan.
6. Place a baking pan on the oven rack. Set to air fry at 400 F for 15 minutes.
7. Serve and enjoy.
Nutrition Info: Calories 120 Fat 5.4 g Carbohydrates 17.1 g Sugar 1.3 g Protein 1.9 g Cholesterol 0 mg

423.Plum Cake

Servings: 8
Cooking Time: 30 Minutes
Ingredients:
- ½ cup butter, soft
- 3 eggs
- ½ cup swerve
- ¼ teaspoon almond extract
- 1 tablespoon vanilla extract
- 1 and ½ cups almond flour
- ½ cup coconut flour
- 2 teaspoons baking powder
- ¾ cup almond milk
- 4 plums, pitted and chopped

Directions:
1. In a bowl, mix all the ingredients and whisk well.
2. Pour this into a cake pan that fits the air fryer after you've lined it with parchment paper, put the pan in the machine and cook at 370 degrees F for 30 minutes.
3. Cool the cake down, slice and serve.
Nutrition Info: calories 183, fat 4, fiber 3, carbs 4, protein 7

424.Currant Cookies

Servings: 6
Cooking Time: 15 Minutes
Ingredients:
- ½ cup currants
- ½ cup swerve
- 2 cups almond flour
- ½ cup ghee; melted
- 1 tsp. vanilla extract
- 2 tsp. baking soda

Directions:
1. Take a bowl and mix all the ingredients and whisk well.
2. Spread this on a baking sheet lined with parchment paper, put the pan in the air fryer and cook at 350°F for 30 minutes
3. Cool down; cut into rectangles and serve.
Nutrition Info: Calories: 172; Fat: 5g; Fiber: 2g; Carbs: 3g; Protein: 5g

425.Honey Hazelnut Apples

Servings: 4
Cooking Time: 13 Minutes
Ingredients:
- 4 apples
- 1 oz butter
- 2 oz breadcrumbs
- Zest of 1 orange
- 2 tbsp chopped hazelnuts
- 2 oz mixed seeds
- 1 tsp cinnamon
- 2 tbsp honey

Directions:
1. Preheat on Bake function to 350 F. Core the apples. Make sure to also score their skin to prevent from splitting. Combine the remaining ingredients in a bowl; stuff the apples with the mixture and cook for 10 minutes. Serve topped with chopped hazelnuts.

426.Fudge Pie

Servings: 8
Cooking Time: 26 Minutes
Ingredients:
- 1½ cups sugar
- ½ cup self-rising flour
- $^1/_3$ cup unsweetened cocoa powder
- 3 large eggs, beaten
- 12 tablespoons (1½ sticks) butter, melted
- 1½ teaspoons vanilla extract
- 1 (9-inch) unbaked pie crust
- ¼ cup confectioners' sugar (optional)

Directions:
1. Thoroughly combine the sugar, flour, and cocoa powder in a medium bowl. Add the beaten eggs and butter and whisk to combine. Stir in the vanilla.
2. Pour the prepared filling into the pie crust and transfer to the baking pan.
3. Slide the baking pan into Rack Position 1, select Convection Bake, set temperature to 350ºF (180ºC), and set time to 26 minutes.
4. When cooking is complete, the pie should be set.
5. Allow the pie to cool for 5 minutes. Sprinkle with the confectioners' sugar, if desired. Serve warm.

427.Garlicky Roasted Mushrooms

Servings: 4
Cooking Time: 27 Minutes
Ingredients:
- 16 garlic cloves, peeled
- 2 teaspoons olive oil, divided
- 16 button mushrooms
- ½ teaspoon dried marjoram
- ⅛ teaspoon freshly ground black pepper
- 1 tablespoon white wine

Directions:
1. Place the garlic cloves in the baking pan and drizzle with 1 teaspoon of the olive oil. Toss to coat well.
2. Slide the baking pan into Rack Position 2, select Roast, set temperature to 350ºF (180ºC) and set time to 12 minutes.

3.   When cooking is complete, remove from the oven. Stir in the mushrooms, marjoram and pepper. Drizzle with the remaining 1 teaspoon of the olive oil and the white wine. Toss to coat well. Return the pan to the oven.
4.   Select Roast, set temperature to 350ºF (180ºC) and set time to 15 minutes.
5.   Once done, the mushrooms and garlic cloves will be softened. Remove from the oven.
6.   Serve warm.

428.Cripsy Artichoke Bites

Servings: 4
Cooking Time: 8 Minutes
Ingredients:
- 14 whole artichoke hearts packed in water
- ½ cup all-purpose flour
- 1 egg
- $^1/_3$ cup panko bread crumbs
- 1 teaspoon Italian seasoning
- Cooking spray

Directions:
1.   Drain the artichoke hearts and dry thoroughly with paper towels.
2.   Place the flour on a plate. Beat the egg in a shallow bowl until frothy. Thoroughly combine the bread crumbs and Italian seasoning in a separate shallow bowl.
3.   Dredge the artichoke hearts in the flour, then in the beaten egg, and finally roll in the bread crumb mixture until evenly coated.
4.   Place the artichoke hearts in the air fryer basket and mist them with cooking spray.
5.   Put the air fryer basket on the baking pan and slide into Rack Position 2, select Air Fry, set temperature to 375ºF (190ºC), and set time to 8 minutes.
6.   Flip the artichoke hearts halfway through the cooking time.
7.   When cooking is complete, the artichoke hearts should start to brown and the edges should be crispy. Remove from the oven and let the artichoke hearts sit for 5 minutes before serving.

429.Baked Peaches And Blueberries

Servings: 6
Cooking Time: 10 Minutes
Ingredients:
- 3 peaches, peeled, halved, and pitted
- 2 tablespoons packed brown sugar
- 1 cup plain Greek yogurt
- ¼ teaspoon ground cinnamon
- 1 teaspoon pure vanilla extract
- 1 cup fresh blueberries

Directions:
1.   Place the peaches in the baking pan, cut-side up. Top with a generous sprinkle of brown sugar.
2.   Slide the baking pan into Rack Position 1, select Convection Bake, set temperature to 380ºF (193ºC), and set time to 10 minutes.
3.   Meanwhile, whisk together the yogurt, cinnamon, and vanilla in a small bowl until smooth.
4.   When cooking is complete, the peaches should be lightly browned and caramelized.
5.   Remove the peaches from the oven to a plate. Serve topped with the yogurt mixture and fresh blueberries.

430.Cheese-stuffed Mushrooms With Pimientos

Servings: 12
Cooking Time: 18 Minutes
Ingredients:
- 24 medium raw white button mushrooms, rinsed and drained
- 4 ounces (113 g) shredded extra-sharp Cheddar cheese
- 2 ounces (57 g) cream cheese, at room temperature
- 1 ounce (28 g) chopped jarred pimientos
- 2 tablespoons grated onion
- ⅛ teaspoon smoked paprika
- ⅛ teaspoon hot sauce
- 2 tablespoons butter, melted, divided
- $^1/_3$ cup panko bread crumbs
- 2 tablespoons grated Parmesan cheese

Directions:
1.   Gently pull out the stems of the mushrooms and discard. Set aside.
2.   In a medium bowl, stir together the Cheddar cheese, cream cheese, pimientos, onion, paprika and hot sauce.
3.   Brush the baking pan with 1 tablespoon of the melted butter. Arrange the mushrooms evenly on the pan, hollow-side up.
4.   Place the cheese mixture into a large heavy plastic bag and cut off the end. Fill the mushrooms with the cheese mixture.
5.   In a small bowl, whisk together the remaining 1 tablespoon of the melted butter, bread crumbs and Parmesan cheese. Sprinkle the panko mixture over each mushroom.
6.   Slide the baking pan into Rack Position 2, select Roast, set temperature to 350ºF (180ºC) and set time to 18 minutes.
7.   When cooking is complete, let the stuffed mushrooms rest for 2 minutes before serving.

431.Crispy Asian Green Beans

Ingredients:
- ½ tsp toasted sesame oil
- 1 tsp peanut oil
- 1-pound green beans, ends trimmed
- 2 cloves garlics, minced
- Coarse sea salt, to taste

Directions:
1. Heat oven on medium heat and add peanut oil until it shimmers.
2. Add garlic and cook about 30 seconds.
3. Add green beans and salt to the pan and roast until golden brown. I
4. At the last minute of cooking, drizzle on toasted sesame oil.

432.Strawberry And Rhubarb Crumble

Servings: 6
Cooking Time: 12 To 17 Minutes
Ingredients:
- 1½ cups sliced fresh strawberries
- $^1/_3$ cup sugar
- ¾ cup sliced rhubarb
- $^2/_3$ cup quick-cooking oatmeal
- ¼ cup packed brown sugar
- ½ cup whole-wheat pastry flour
- ½ teaspoon ground cinnamon
- 3 tablespoons unsalted butter, melted

Directions:
1. Place the strawberries, sugar, and rhubarb in the baking pan and toss to coat.
2. Combine the oatmeal, brown sugar, pastry flour, and cinnamon in a medium bowl.
3. Add the melted butter to the oatmeal mixture and stir until crumbly. Sprinkle this generously on top of the strawberries and rhubarb.
4. Slide the baking pan into Rack Position 1, select Convection Bake, set temperature to 370ºF (188ºC), and set the time to 12 minutes.
5. Bake until the fruit is bubbly and the topping is golden brown. Continue cooking for an additional 2 to 5 minutes if needed.
6. When cooking is complete, remove from the oven and serve warm.

433.Apple Treat With Raisins

Servings: 4
Cooking Time: 15 Minutes
Ingredients:
- 4 apples, cored
- 1 ½ oz almonds
- ¾ oz raisins
- 2 tbsp sugar

Directions:
1. Preheat Breville on Bake function to 360 F. In a bowl, mix sugar, almonds, and raisins and blend the mixture using a hand mixer. Fill cored apples with the almond mixture. Place the prepared apples in the basket and press Start. Bake for 10 minutes. Serve with powdered sugar.

434.Blueberry Apple Crumble

Servings: 6
Cooking Time: 15 Minutes
Ingredients:
- 1 medium apple, finely diced
- 1/2 cup of frozen blueberries strawberries
- 2/3 cup of rice flour
- 2 tablespoons of sugar
- 1/2 teaspoon of ground cinnamon
- 2 tablespoons of nondairy butter

Directions:
1. Set the Instant Vortex on Air fryer to 350 degrees F for 15 minutes. Combine apple with blueberries in a bowl. Mingle butter with flour, cinnamon, and sugar in another bowl. Pour the butter mixture into the apple mixture. Transfer this mixture on the cooking tray. Insert the cooking tray in the Vortex when it displays "Add Food". Flip the sides when it displays "Turn Food". Remove from the oven when cooking time is complete. Serve warm.
Nutrition Info: Calories: 379 Cal Total Fat: 29.7 g Saturated Fat: 0 g Cholesterol: 0 mg Sodium: 0 mg Total Carbs: 23.7 g Fiber: 0 g Sugar: 0 g Protein: 5.2 g

435.Berry Tacos

Servings: 2
Cooking Time: 5 Minutes
Ingredients:
- 2 soft shell tortillas
- 4 tablespoons strawberry jelly
- ¼ cup fresh blueberries
- ¼ cup fresh raspberries
- 2 tablespoons powdered sugar

Directions:
1. Spread 2 tablespoons of strawberry jelly over each tortilla
2. Top each with berries evenly and sprinkle with powdered sugar.
3. Press "Power Button" of Air Fry Oven and turn the dial to select the "Air Fry" mode.
4. Press the Time button and again turn the dial to set the cooking time to 5 minutes.

5. Now push the Temp button and rotate the dial to set the temperature at 300 degrees F.
6. Press "Start/Pause" button to start.
7. When the unit beeps to show that it is preheated, open the lid.
8. Arrange the tortillas in "Air Fry Basket" and insert in the oven.
9. Serve warm.

Nutrition Info: Calories 216 Total Fat 0.8 g Saturated Fat 0.1 g Cholesterol 0mg Sodium 11 mg Total Carbs 53.2 g Fiber 3 g Sugar 38.7 g Protein 1.7 g

436.Chocolate Donuts

Servings: 8-10
Cooking Time: 20 Minutes
Ingredients:
- (8-ounce) can jumbo biscuits
- Cooking oil
- Chocolate sauce, such as Hershey's

Directions:
1. Preparing the Ingredients. Separate the biscuit dough into 8 biscuits and place them on a flat work surface. Use a small circle cookie cutter or a biscuit cutter to cut a hole in the center of each biscuit. You can also cut the holes using a knife.
2. Spray the Oven rack/basket with cooking oil. Place the Rack on the middle-shelf of the air fryer oven.
3. Air Frying. Place 4 donuts in the air fryer oven. Do not stack. Spray with cooking oil. Cook for 4 minutes.
4. Open the air fryer oven and flip the donuts. Cook for an additional 4 minutes.
5. Remove the cooked donuts from the air fryer, then repeat steps 3 and 4 for the remaining 4 donuts.
6. Drizzle chocolate sauce over the donuts and enjoy while warm.

Nutrition Info: CALORIES: 181; FAT:98G; PROTEIN:3G; FIBER:1G

437.Strawberry Tart

Ingredients:
- 2 cups sliced strawberries
- 1 cup fresh cream
- 3 tbsp. butter
- 1 ½ cup plain flour
- 3 tbsp. unsalted butter
- 2 tbsp. powdered sugar
- 2 cups cold water

Directions:
1. In a large bowl, mix the flour, cocoa powder, butter and sugar with your Oregano Fingers. The mixture should resemble breadcrumbs. Squeeze the

dough using the cold milk and wrap it and leave it to cool for ten minutes. Roll the dough out into the pie and prick the sides of the pie.
2. Mix the ingredients for the filling in a bowl. Make sure that it is a little
3. thick. Preheat the fryer to 300 Fahrenheit for five minutes. You will need to place the tin in the basket and cover it. When the pastry has turned golden brown, you will need to remove the tin and let it cool. Cut into slices and serve with a dollop of cream.

438.Garlicky-lemon Zucchini

Ingredients:
- Coarse salt and black pepper, to taste
- ½ tsp thyme, minced
- ½ lemon
- 4 small green zucchinis, any color, sliced about ¼-inch thick
- 1½ Tbsp extra virgin olive oil
- 1 Tbsp garlic, minced

Directions:
1. Heat oven over medium-low heat. Add oil and let heat for 1 minute.
2. Sprinkle zucchini with salt and pepper.
3. Add to the pan in a single layer. When zucchini is nicely browned, flip
4. and brown on other side.
5. Add garlic and saute for 1 minute.
6. Sprinkle thyme and additional salt if necessary.
7. Remove from pan and squeeze lemon juice on zucchini.

439.Banana S'mores

Servings: 4
Cooking Time: 4 Minutes
Ingredients:
- 4 bananas
- 3 tablespoons of mini semi-sweet chocolate chips
- 3 tablespoons of mini marshmallows
- 3 tablespoons of graham cracker cereal
- Aluminum foil
- Cooking oil spray

Directions:
1. Set the Instant Vortex on Air fryer to 350 degrees F for 4 minutes. Place the bananas on the aluminum foil sheet greased with cooking oil spray. Tear open the banana from one side to form a pocket. Top with the chocolate chips, marshmallows, and graham cracker cereal. Cover completely with foil and place on the cooking tray. Insert the cooking tray in the Vortex when it displays "Add Food". Remove

from the oven when cooking time is complete. Serve warm.

Nutrition Info: Calories: 249 Cal Total Fat: 11.9 g Saturated Fat: 0 g Cholesterol: 0 mg Sodium: 0 mg Total Carbs: 14.8 g Fiber: 0 g Sugar: 0 g Protein: 5 g

440.Sago Payada

Ingredients:
- 3 tbsp. powdered sugar
- 3 tbsp. unsalted butter
- 2 cups milk
- 2 cups-soaked sago
- 2 tbsp. custard powder

Directions:
1. Boil the milk and the sugar in a pan and add the custard powder followed by the sago and stir till you get a thick mixture.
2. Preheat the fryer to 300 Fahrenheit for five minutes. Place the dish in the basket and reduce the temperature to 250 Fahrenheit. Cook for ten minutes and set aside to cool.

441.Nutella Banana Muffins

Servings: 12
Cooking Time: 25 Minutes
Ingredients:
- 1 2/3 cups plain flour
- 1 teaspoon baking soda
- 1 teaspoon baking powder
- 1 teaspoon ground cinnamon
- ¼ teaspoon salt
- 4 ripe bananas, peeled and mashed
- 2 eggs
- ½ cup brown sugar
- 1 teaspoon vanilla essence
- 3 tablespoons milk
- 1 tablespoon Nutella
- ¼ cup walnuts

Directions:
1. Grease 12 muffin molds. Set aside.
2. In a large bowl, sift together the flour, baking soda, baking powder, cinnamon, and salt.
3. In another bowl, mix together the remaining ingredients except walnuts.
4. Add the banana mixture into flour mixture and mix until just combined.
5. Fold in the walnuts.
6. Place the mixture into the prepared muffin molds.
7. Press "Power Button" of Air Fry Oven and turn the dial to select the "Air Fry" mode.
8. Press the Time button and again turn the dial to set the cooking time to 25 minutes.

9. Now push the Temp button and rotate the dial to set the temperature at 250 degrees F.
10. Press "Start/Pause" button to start.
11. When the unit beeps to show that it is preheated, open the lid.
12. Arrange the muffin molds in "Air Fry Basket" and insert in the oven.
13. Place the muffin molds onto a wire rack to cool for about 10 minutes.
14. Carefully, invert the muffins onto the wire rack to completely cool before serving.

Nutrition Info: Calories 227 Total Fat 6.6 g Saturated Fat 1.5 g Cholesterol 45 mg Sodium 221 mg Total Carbs 38.1 g Fiber 2.4 g Sugar 15.8 g Protein 5.2 g

442.Polenta Fries With Chili-lime Mayo

Servings: 4
Cooking Time: 28 Minutes
Ingredients:
- Polenta Fries:
- 2 teaspoons vegetable or olive oil
- ¼ teaspoon paprika
- 1 pound (454 g) prepared polenta, cut into 3-inch × ½-inch strips
- Salt and freshly ground black pepper, to taste
- Chili-Lime Mayo:
- ½ cup mayonnaise
- 1 teaspoon chili powder
- 1 teaspoon chopped fresh cilantro
- ¼ teaspoon ground cumin
- Juice of ½ lime
- Salt and freshly ground black pepper, to taste

Directions:
1. Mix the oil and paprika in a bowl. Add the polenta strips and toss until evenly coated. Transfer the polenta strips to the air fryer basket.
2. Put the air fryer basket on the baking pan and slide into Rack Position 2, select Air Fry, set temperature to 400ºF (205ºC), and set time to 28 minutes.
3. Stir the polenta strips halfway through the cooking time.
4. Meanwhile, whisk together all the ingredients for the chili-lime mayo in a small bowl.
5. When cooking is complete, remove the polenta fries from the oven to a plate. Season as desired with salt and pepper. Serve alongside the chili-lime mayo as a dipping sauce.

443.Vanilla Brownie Squares

Servings: 2
Cooking Time: 25 Minutes

Ingredients:
- 1 whole egg, beaten
- ¼ cup chocolate chips
- 2 tbsp white sugar
- ⅓ cup flour
- 2 tbsp safflower oil
- 1 tsp vanilla
- ¼ cup cocoa powder

Directions:
1. Preheat on Bake function to 360 F. In a bowl, mix the egg, sugar, olive oil, and vanilla. In another bowl, mix cocoa powder and flour. Add the flour mixture to the vanilla mixture and stir until fully incorporated.
2. Pour the mixture into a greased baking pan and sprinkle chocolate chips on top. Cook for 20 minutes. Chill and cut into squares to serve.

444.Mixed Berries With Pecan Streusel

Servings: 3
Cooking Time: 15 Minutes
Ingredients:
- 3 tablespoons pecans, chopped
- 3 tablespoons almonds, slivered
- 2 tablespoons walnuts, chopped
- 3 tablespoons granulated swerve
- 1/2 teaspoon ground cinnamon
- 1 egg
- 2 tablespoons cold salted butter, cut into pieces
- 1/2 cup mixed berries

Directions:
1. Mix your nuts, swerve, cinnamon, egg, and butter until well combined.
2. Place mixed berries on the bottom of a lightly greased Air Fryer-safe dish. Top with the prepared topping.
3. Bake at 340 degrees F for 17 minutes. Serve at room temperature.
Nutrition Info: 255 Calories; 28g Fat; 1g Carbs; 3g Protein; 6g Sugars; 4g FiberEasy Fluffy Pancakes

445.Nutella Banana Pastries

Servings: 4
Cooking Time: 12 Minutes
Ingredients:
- 1 puff pastry sheet
- ½ cup Nutella
- 2 bananas, peeled and sliced

Directions:
1. Cut the pastry sheet into 4 equal-sized squares.
2. Spread the Nutella on each square of pastry evenly.
3. Divide the banana slices over Nutella.

4. Fold each square into a triangle and with wet fingers, slightly press the edges.
5. Then with a fork, press the edges firmly.
6. Press "Power Button" of Air Fry Oven and turn the dial to select the "Air Fry" mode.
7. Press the Time button and again turn the dial to set the cooking time to 12 minutes.
8. Now push the Temp button and rotate the dial to set the temperature at 375 degrees F.
9. Press "Start/Pause" button to start.
10. When the unit beeps to show that it is preheated, open the lid.
11. Arrange the pastries in greased "Air Fry Basket" and insert in the oven.
12. Serve warm.
Nutrition Info: Calories 221 Total Fat 10 g Saturated Fat 2.7 g Cholesterol 26 mg Sodium 103 mg Total Carbs 31.6 g Fiber 2.6 g Sugar 14.4 g Protein 3.4 g

446.Crustless Pizza

Servings: 1
Cooking Time: 15 Minutes
Ingredients:
- 2 slices sugar-free bacon; cooked and crumbled
- 7 slices pepperoni
- ½ cup shredded mozzarella cheese
- ¼ cup cooked ground sausage
- 2 tbsp. low-carb, sugar-free pizza sauce, for dipping
- 1 tbsp. grated Parmesan cheese

Directions:
1. Cover the bottom of a 6-inch cake pan with mozzarella. Place pepperoni, sausage and bacon on top of cheese and sprinkle with Parmesan
2. Place pan into the air fryer basket. Adjust the temperature to 400 Degrees F and set the timer for 5 minutes.
3. Remove when cheese is bubbling and golden. Serve warm with pizza sauce for dipping.
Nutrition Info: Calories: 466; Protein: 21g; Fiber: 5g; Fat: 30g; Carbs: 2g

447.Almond Flour Blackberry Muffins

Servings: 8
Cooking Time: 12 Minutes
Ingredients:
- ½ cup fresh blackberries
- Dry Ingredients:
- 1½ cups almond flour
- 1 teaspoon baking powder
- ½ teaspoon baking soda
- ½ cup Swerve
- ¼ teaspoon kosher salt

- Wet Ingredients:
- 2 eggs
- ¼ cup coconut oil, melted
- ½ cup milk
- ½ teaspoon vanilla paste

Directions:
1. Line an 8-cup muffin tin with paper liners.
2. Thoroughly combine the almond flour, baking powder, baking soda, Swerve, and salt in a mixing bowl.
3. Whisk together the eggs, coconut oil, milk, and vanilla in a separate mixing bowl until smooth.
4. Add the wet mixture to the dry and fold in the blackberries. Stir with a spatula just until well incorporated.
5. Spoon the batter into the prepared muffin cups, filling each about three-quarters full.
6. Put the muffin tin into Rack Position 1, select Convection Bake, set temperature to 350ºF (180ºC), and set time to 12 minutes.
7. When done, the tops should be golden and a toothpick inserted in the middle should come out clean.
8. Allow the muffins to cool in the muffin tin for 10 minutes before removing and serving

448.Crispy Eggplant Bites

Servings: 4
Cooking Time: 20 Minutes
Ingredients:
- 1 eggplant, cut into 1-inch pieces
- 1 tsp garlic powder
- 2 tbsp olive oil
- 1/2 tsp Italian seasoning
- 1 tsp paprika
- 1/2 tsp red pepper

Directions:
1. Fit the oven with the rack in position 2.
2. Add all ingredients into the large mixing bowl and toss well.
3. Transfer eggplant mixture in air fryer basket then places air fryer basket in baking pan.
4. Place a baking pan on the oven rack. Set to air fry at 375 F for 20 minutes.
5. Serve and enjoy.
Nutrition Info: Calories 99 Fat 7.5 g Carbohydrates 8.7 g Sugar 4.5 g Protein 1.5 g Cholesterol 0 mg

449.Air Fryer Nuts

Servings: 4
Cooking Time: 9 Minutes
Ingredients:
- 1/2 cup macadamia nuts

- 1/4 cup walnuts
- 1/4 cup hazelnuts
- 1/2 cup pecans
- 1 tbsp olive oil
- 1 tsp salt

Directions:
1. Fit the oven with the rack in position 2.
2. Add all nuts to the air fryer basket then place an air fryer basket in the baking pan.
3. Place a baking pan on the oven rack. Set to air fry at 320 F for 9 minutes.
4. Drizzle nuts with olive oil and season with salt and toss well.
5. Serve and enjoy.
Nutrition Info: Calories 280 Fat 29 g Carbohydrates 4.9 g Sugar 1.3 g Protein 4.7 g Cholesterol 0 mg

450.Three Berry Crumble

Ingredients:
- ¾ cup brown sugar
- ¾ cup old fashioned oats
- ½ cup chopped almonds
- 1 tsp cinnamon
- 6 cups of fresh mixed berries (blueberries, raspberries), washed and dried
- ¼ cup sugar
- ¼ cup flour
- 1 Tbsp lemon juice
- ¾ cup flour
- 1 stick cold butter, cut into cubes

Directions:
1. Preheat oven to 375°F.
2. Lightly toss the berries, sugar, flour and lemon juice inside your oven.
3. In a bowl, mix the flour, brown sugar, oats, almonds and cinnamon.
4. Incorporate cold butter with your fingertips into the oat mixture until small clumps form.
5. Pour topping onto fruit and bake for 45 minutes to 1 hour, until bubbles form and top appears browned and crispy.
6. Serve with vanilla ice cream right out of oven.

451.Buttermilk Biscuits

Ingredients:
- 4 tsp baking powder
- ¼ tsp baking soda
- ¼ tsp salt
- 4 Tbsp softened butter
- 1 cup all-purpose flour
- 1 cup whole wheat flour
- 2 Tbsp sugar
- 1¼ cups cold buttermilk

Directions:
1. Preheat oven to 400°F.
2. In a bowl, combine flours, sugar, baking powder, baking soda and salt.
3. Add softened butter and use your Oregano Fingers to work the butter into the flour until the mixture resembles coarse crumbs.
4. Stir in the buttermilk, forming a soft dough.
5. Turn the dough onto a floured surface and pat into a ¾ inch thick circle.
6. With a 2-inch biscuit cutter, cut out biscuits, gathering dough as needed to shape more biscuits.
7. Arrange biscuits in oven and bake until golden brown, about 12 minutes.

452. Sweet And Sour Meatballs

Ingredients:
- ¼ cup apple cider vinegar
- 1 (10-ounce) can condensed tomato soup
- cup sugar
- 1 (8-ounce) can pineapple tidbits, undrained
- 1-pound ground beef
- 1 egg
- ½ cup grated Parmesan cheese
- ¼ cup dry bread crumbs

Directions:
1. Preheat oven to 350ºF. In medium bowl, combine ground beef, egg, cheese, and bread crumbs and mix well to blend. Form into 1-inch meatballs and place on baking sheet. Bake at 350°F for 20 to 25 minutes or until no longer pink in center. Chill meatballs in refrigerator until thoroughly cold.
2. In a medium bowl, combine vinegar, soup, sugar, and pineapple tidbits and juice. Mix well and pour into 1-gallon-size zipper-lock freezer bag. Add meatballs, seal bag, and turn gently to mix. Label bag and freeze.
3. To thaw and reheat: Thaw overnight in refrigerator. Pour meatballs and sauce into large skillet and cook over medium heat until sauce comes to a boil. Reduce heat, cover, and simmer meatballs for 8 to 10 minutes or until thoroughly heated, stirring occasionally.

453. Tomatoes Dip

Servings: 6
Cooking Time: 15 Minutes
Ingredients:
- 12 oz. cream cheese, soft
- 8 oz. mozzarella cheese; grated
- ¼ cup basil; chopped.
- ¼ cup parmesan; grated
- 4 garlic cloves; minced

- 1 pint grape tomatoes; halved
- 2 tbsp. thyme; chopped.
- ½ tbsp. oregano; chopped.
- 1 tsp. olive oil
- A pinch of salt and black pepper

Directions:
1. Put the tomatoes in your air fryer's basket and cook them at 400°F for 15 minutes.
2. In a blender, combine the fried tomatoes with the rest of the ingredients and pulse well
3. Transfer this to a ramekin, place it in the air fryer and cook at 400°F for 5 - 6 minutes more. Serve as a snack

Nutrition Info: Calories: 184; Fat: 8g; Fiber: 3g; Carbs: 4g; Protein: 8g

454. Raspberry Cream Rol-ups

Servings: 4
Cooking Time: 25 Minutes
Ingredients:
- 1 cup of fresh raspberries rinsed and patted dry
- ½ cup of cream cheese softened to room temperature
- ¼ cup of brown sugar
- ¼ cup of sweetened condensed milk
- 1 egg
- 1 teaspoon of corn starch
- 6 spring roll wrappers (any brand will do, we like Blue Dragon or Tasty Joy, both available through Target or Walmart, or any large grocery chain)
- ¼ cup of water

Directions:
1. Preparing the Ingredients. Cover the basket of the air fryer oven with a lining of tin foil, leaving the edges uncovered to allow air to circulate through the basket. Preheat the air fryer oven to 350 degrees.
2. In a mixing bowl, combine the cream cheese, brown sugar, condensed milk, cornstarch, and egg. Beat or whip thoroughly, until all ingredients are completely mixed and fluffy, thick and stiff.
3. Spoon even amounts of the creamy filling into each spring roll wrapper, then top each dollop of filling with several raspberries.
4. Roll up the wraps around the creamy raspberry filling, and seal the seams with a few dabs of water.
5. Place each roll on the foil-lined Oven rack/basket, seams facing down. Place the Rack on the middle-shelf of the air fryer oven.
6. Air Frying. Set the air fryer oven timer to 10 minutes. During cooking, shake the handle of the fryer basket to ensure a nice even surface crisp.
7. After 10 minutes, when the air fryer oven shuts off, the spring rolls should be golden brown and perfect on the outside, while the raspberries and

cream filling will have cooked together in a glorious fusion. Remove with tongs and serve hot or cold.

455.Cheesy Sweet Pepper Poppers

Servings: 10
Cooking Time: 15 Minutes
Ingredients:
- 2 tbsp cilantro, chopped
- 8 oz cream cheese
- 8 oz gouda cheese, grated
- 1 lb mini sweet peppers, halved
- 2 garlic cloves, minced
- 1/4 cup onion, grated
- 1/2 cup feta cheese, crumbled

Directions:
1. Fit the oven with the rack in position
2. Add all ingredients except peppers into the bowl and mix well to combine.
3. Stuff each pepper halves with cheese mixture and place in baking pan.
4. Set to bake at 425 F for 20 minutes. After 5 minutes place the baking pan in the preheated oven.
5. Serve and enjoy.

Nutrition Info: Calories 186 Fat 15.8 g Carbohydrates 2.8 g Sugar 1.6 g Protein 8.6 g Cholesterol 57 mg

456.Spiced Apple Chips

Servings: 4
Cooking Time: 10 Minutes
Ingredients:
- 4 medium apples (any type will work), cored and thinly sliced
- ¼ teaspoon nutmeg
- ¼ teaspoon cinnamon
- Cooking spray

Directions:
1. Place the apple slices in a large bowl and sprinkle the spices on top. Toss to coat.
2. Put the apple slices in the air fryer basket in a single layer and spray them with cooking spray.
3. Put the air fryer basket on the baking pan and slide into Rack Position 2, select Air Fry, set temperature to 360ºF (182ºC), and set time to 10 minutes.
4. Stir the apple slices halfway through.
5. When cooking is complete, the apple chips should be crispy. Transfer the apple chips to a paper towel-lined plate and rest for 5 minutes before serving.

OTHER FAVORITE RECIPES

457.Chorizo, Corn, And Potato Frittata

Servings: 4
Cooking Time: 12 Minutes
Ingredients:
- 2 tablespoons olive oil
- 1 chorizo, sliced
- 4 eggs
- ½ cup corn
- 1 large potato, boiled and cubed
- 1 tablespoon chopped parsley
- ½ cup feta cheese, crumbled
- Salt and ground black pepper, to taste

Directions:
1. Heat the olive oil in a nonstick skillet over medium heat until shimmering.
2. Add the chorizo and cook for 4 minutes or until golden brown.
3. Whisk the eggs in a bowl, then sprinkle with salt and ground black pepper.
4. Mix the remaining ingredients in the egg mixture, then pour the chorizo and its fat into the baking pan. Pour in the egg mixture.
5. Slide the baking pan into Rack Position 1, select Convection Bake, set temperature to 330ºF (166ºC) and set time to 8 minutes.
6. Stir the mixture halfway through.
7. When cooking is complete, the eggs should be set.
8. Serve immediately.

458.Taco Beef And Chile Casserole

Servings: 4
Cooking Time: 15 Minutes
Ingredients:
- 1 pound (454 g) 85% lean ground beef
- 1 tablespoon taco seasoning
- 1 (7-ounce / 198-g) can diced mild green chiles
- ½ cup milk
- 2 large eggs
- 1 cup shredded Mexican cheese blend
- 2 tablespoons all-purpose flour
- ½ teaspoon kosher salt
- Cooking spray

Directions:
1. Spritz the baking pan with cooking spray.
2. Toss the ground beef with taco seasoning in a large bowl to mix well. Pour the seasoned ground beef in the prepared baking pan.
3. Combing the remaining ingredients in a medium bowl. Whisk to mix well, then pour the mixture over the ground beef.

4. Slide the baking pan into Rack Position 1, select Convection Bake, set temperature to 350ºF (180ºC) and set time to 15 minutes.
5. When cooking is complete, a toothpick inserted in the center should come out clean.
6. Remove the casserole from the oven and allow to cool for 5 minutes, then slice to serve.

459.Simple Cheesy Shrimps

Servings: 4 To 6
Cooking Time: 8 Minutes
Ingredients:
- $^2/_3$ cup grated Parmesan cheese
- 4 minced garlic cloves
- 1 teaspoon onion powder
- ½ teaspoon oregano
- 1 teaspoon basil
- 1 teaspoon ground black pepper
- 2 tablespoons olive oil
- 2 pounds (907 g) cooked large shrimps, peeled and deveined
- Lemon wedges, for topping
- Cooking spray

Directions:
1. Spritz the air fryer basket with cooking spray.
2. Combine all the ingredients, except for the shrimps, in a large bowl. Stir to mix well.
3. Dunk the shrimps in the mixture and toss to coat well. Shake the excess off. Arrange the shrimps in the basket.
4. Put the air fryer basket on the baking pan and slide into Rack Position 2, select Air Fry, set temperature to 350ºF (180ºC) and set time to 8 minutes.
5. Flip the shrimps halfway through the cooking time.
6. When cooking is complete, the shrimps should be opaque. Transfer the cooked shrimps onto a large plate and squeeze the lemon wedges over before serving.

460.Air Fried Bacon Pinwheels

Servings: 8 Pinwheels
Cooking Time: 10 Minutes
Ingredients:
- 1 sheet puff pastry
- 2 tablespoons maple syrup
- ¼ cup brown sugar
- 8 slices bacon
- Ground black pepper, to taste
- Cooking spray

Directions:

1. Spritz the air fryer basket with cooking spray.
2. Roll the puff pastry into a 10-inch square with a rolling pin on a clean work surface, then cut the pastry into 8 strips.
3. Brush the strips with maple syrup and sprinkle with sugar, leaving a 1-inch far end uncovered.
4. Arrange each slice of bacon on each strip, leaving a ⅛-inch length of bacon hang over the end close to you. Sprinkle with black pepper.
5. From the end close to you, roll the strips into pinwheels, then dab the uncovered end with water and seal the rolls.
6. Arrange the pinwheels in the basket and spritz with cooking spray.
7. Put the air fryer basket on the baking pan and slide into Rack Position 2, select Air Fry, set temperature to 360ºF (182ºC) and set time to 10 minutes.
8. Flip the pinwheels halfway through.
9. When cooking is complete, the pinwheels should be golden brown. Remove from the oven and serve immediately.

461. Goat Cheese And Asparagus Frittata

Servings: 2 To 4
Cooking Time: 25 Minutes
Ingredients:
*   1 cup asparagus spears, cut into 1-inch pieces
*   1 teaspoon vegetable oil
*   1 tablespoon milk
*   6 eggs, beaten
*   2 ounces (57 g) goat cheese, crumbled
*   1 tablespoon minced chives, optional
*   Kosher salt and pepper, to taste
*   Add the asparagus spears to a small bowl and drizzle with the vegetable oil. Toss until well coated and transfer to the air fryer basket.
Directions:
1. Put the air fryer basket on the baking pan and slide into Rack Position 2, select Air Fry, set temperature to 400ºF (205ºC) and set time to 5 minutes.
2. Flip the asparagus halfway through.
3. When cooking is complete, the asparagus should be tender and slightly wilted.
4. Remove from the oven to the baking pan.
5. Stir together the milk and eggs in a medium bowl. Pour the mixture over the asparagus in the pan. Sprinkle with the goat cheese and the chives (if using) over the eggs. Season with salt and pepper.
6. Slide the baking pan into Rack Position 1, select Convection Bake, set temperature to 320ºF (160ºC) and set time to 20 minutes.
7. When cooking is complete, the top should be golden and the eggs should be set.

8. Transfer to a serving dish. Slice and serve.

462. Potato Chips With Lemony Cream Dip

Servings: 2 To 4
Cooking Time: 15 Minutes
Ingredients:
*   2 large russet potatoes, sliced into ⅛-inch slices, rinsed
*   Sea salt and freshly ground black pepper, to taste
*   Cooking spray
*   Lemony Cream Dip:
*   ½ cup sour cream
*   ¼ teaspoon lemon juice
*   2 scallions, white part only, minced
*   1 tablespoon olive oil
*   ¼ teaspoon salt
*   Freshly ground black pepper, to taste
Directions:
1. Soak the potato slices in water for 10 minutes, then pat dry with paper towels.
2. Transfer the potato slices in the air fryer basket. Spritz the slices with cooking spray.
3. Put the air fryer basket on the baking pan and slide into Rack Position 2, select Air Fry, set temperature to 300ºF (150ºC) and set time to 15 minutes.
4. Stir the potato slices three times during cooking. Sprinkle with salt and ground black pepper in the last minute.
5. Meanwhile, combine the ingredients for the dip in a small bowl. Stir to mix well.
6. When cooking is complete, the potato slices will be crispy and golden brown. Remove from the oven and serve the potato chips immediately with the dip.

463. Lemony And Garlicky Asparagus

Servings: 10 Spears
Cooking Time: 10 Minutes
Ingredients:
*   10 spears asparagus (about ½ pound / 227 g in total), snap the ends off
*   1 tablespoon lemon juice
*   2 teaspoons minced garlic
*   ½ teaspoon salt
*   ¼ teaspoon ground black pepper
*   Cooking spray
Directions:
1. Line the air fryer basket with parchment paper.
2. Put the asparagus spears in a large bowl. Drizzle with lemon juice and sprinkle with minced garlic, salt, and ground black pepper. Toss to coat well.

3. Transfer the asparagus to the basket and spritz with cooking spray.
4. Put the air fryer basket on the baking pan and slide into Rack Position 2, select Air Fry, set temperature to 400ºF (205ºC) and set time to 10 minutes.
5. Flip the asparagus halfway through cooking.
6. When cooked, the asparagus should be wilted and soft. Remove from the oven and serve immediately.

464. Salty Tortilla Chips

Servings: 4
Cooking Time: 10 Minutes
Ingredients:
- 4 six-inch corn tortillas, cut in half and slice into thirds
- 1 tablespoon canola oil
- ¼ teaspoon kosher salt
- Cooking spray

Directions:
1. Spritz the air fryer basket with cooking spray.
2. On a clean work surface, brush the tortilla chips with canola oil, then transfer the chips to the basket.
3. Put the air fryer basket on the baking pan and slide into Rack Position 2, select Air Fry, set temperature to 360ºF (182ºC) and set time to 10 minutes.
4. Flip the chips and sprinkle with salt halfway through the cooking time.
5. When cooked, the chips will be crunchy and lightly browned. Transfer the chips to a plate lined with paper towels. Serve immediately.

465. Fast Cinnamon Toast

Servings: 6
Cooking Time: 5 Minutes
Ingredients:
- 1½ teaspoons cinnamon
- 1½ teaspoons vanilla extract
- ½ cup sugar
- 2 teaspoons ground black pepper
- 2 tablespoons melted coconut oil
- 12 slices whole wheat bread

Directions:
1. Combine all the ingredients, except for the bread, in a large bowl. Stir to mix well.
2. Dunk the bread in the bowl of mixture gently to coat and infuse well. Shake the excess off. Arrange the bread slices in the air fryer basket.
3. Put the air fryer basket on the baking pan and slide into Rack Position 2, select Air Fry, set

temperature to 400ºF (205ºC) and set time to 5 minutes.
4. Flip the bread halfway through.
5. When cooking is complete, the bread should be golden brown.
6. Remove the bread slices from the oven and slice to serve.

466. Keto Cheese Quiche

Servings: 8
Cooking Time: 1 Hour
Ingredients:
- Crust:
- 1¼ cups blanched almond flour
- 1 large egg, beaten
- 1¼ cups grated Parmesan cheese
- ¼ teaspoon fine sea salt
- Filling:
- 4 ounces (113 g) cream cheese
- 1 cup shredded Swiss cheese
- $1/3$ cup minced leeks
- 4 large eggs, beaten
- ½ cup chicken broth
- ⅛ teaspoon cayenne pepper
- ¾ teaspoon fine sea salt
- 1 tablespoon unsalted butter, melted
- Chopped green onions, for garnish
- Cooking spray

Directions:
1. Spritz the baking pan with cooking spray.
2. Combine the flour, egg, Parmesan, and salt in a large bowl. Stir to mix until a satiny and firm dough forms.
3. Arrange the dough between two grease parchment papers, then roll the dough into a $1/16$-inch thick circle.
4. Make the crust: Transfer the dough into the prepared pan and press to coat the bottom.
5. Slide the baking pan into Rack Position 1, select Convection Bake, set temperature to 325ºF (163ºC) and set time to 12 minutes.
6. When cooking is complete, the edges of the crust should be lightly browned.
7. Meanwhile, combine the ingredient for the filling, except for the green onions in a large bowl.
8. Pour the filling over the cooked crust and cover the edges of the crust with aluminum foil.
9. Slide the baking pan into Rack Position 1, select Convection Bake, set time to 15 minutes.
10. When cooking is complete, reduce the heat to 300ºF (150ºC) and set time to 30 minutes.
11. When cooking is complete, a toothpick inserted in the center should come out clean.
12. Remove from the oven and allow to cool for 10 minutes before serving.

467.Chocolate Buttermilk Cake

Servings: 8
Cooking Time: 20 Minutes
Ingredients:
- 1 cup all-purpose flour
- $^2/_3$ cup granulated white sugar
- ¼ cup unsweetened cocoa powder
- ¾ teaspoon baking soda
- ¼ teaspoon salt
- $^2/_3$ cup buttermilk
- 2 tablespoons plus 2 teaspoons vegetable oil
- 1 teaspoon vanilla extract
- Cooking spray

Directions:
1. Spritz the baking pan with cooking spray.
2. Combine the flour, cocoa powder, baking soda, sugar, and salt in a large bowl. Stir to mix well.
3. Mix in the buttermilk, vanilla, and vegetable oil. Keep stirring until it forms a grainy and thick dough.
4. Scrape the chocolate batter from the bowl and transfer to the pan, level the batter in an even layer with a spatula.
5. Slide the baking pan into Rack Position 1, select Convection Bake, set temperature to 325ºF (163ºC) and set time to 20 minutes.
6. After 15 minutes, remove the pan from the oven. Check the doneness. Return the pan to the oven and continue cooking.
7. When done, a toothpick inserted in the center should come out clean.
8. Invert the cake on a cooling rack and allow to cool for 15 minutes before slicing to serve.

468.Corn On The Cob With Mayonnaise

Servings: 4
Cooking Time: 10 Minutes
Ingredients:
- 2 tablespoons mayonnaise
- 2 teaspoons minced garlic
- ½ teaspoon sea salt
- 1 cup panko bread crumbs
- 4 (4-inch length) ears corn on the cob, husk and silk removed
- Cooking spray

Directions:
1. Spritz the air fryer basket with cooking spray.
2. Combine the mayonnaise, garlic, and salt in a bowl. Stir to mix well. Pour the panko on a plate.
3. Brush the corn on the cob with mayonnaise mixture, then roll the cob in the bread crumbs and press to coat well.
4. Transfer the corn on the cob in the basket and spritz with cooking spray.
5. Put the air fryer basket on the baking pan and slide into Rack Position 2, select Air Fry, set temperature to 400ºF (205ºC) and set time to 10 minutes.
6. Flip the corn on the cob at least three times during the cooking.
7. When cooked, the corn kernels on the cob should be almost browned. Remove from the oven and serve immediately.

469.Shrimp With Sriracha And Worcestershire Sauce

Servings: 4
Cooking Time: 10 Minutes
Ingredients:
- 1 tablespoon Sriracha sauce
- 1 teaspoon Worcestershire sauce
- 2 tablespoons sweet chili sauce
- ¾ cup mayonnaise
- 1 egg, beaten
- 1 cup panko bread crumbs
- 1 pound (454 g) raw shrimp, shelled and deveined, rinsed and drained
- Lime wedges, for serving
- Cooking spray

Directions:
1. Spritz the air fryer basket with cooking spray.
2. Combine the Sriracha sauce, Worcestershire sauce, chili sauce, and mayo in a bowl. Stir to mix well. Reserve $^1/_3$ cup of the mixture as the dipping sauce.
3. Combine the remaining sauce mixture with the beaten egg. Stir to mix well. Put the panko in a separate bowl.
4. Dredge the shrimp in the sauce mixture first, then into the panko. Roll the shrimp to coat well. Shake the excess off.
5. Place the shrimp in the basket, then spritz with cooking spray.
6. Put the air fryer basket on the baking pan and slide into Rack Position 2, select Air Fry, set temperature to 360ºF (182ºC) and set time to 10 minutes.
7. Flip the shrimp halfway through the cooking time.
8. When cooking is complete, the shrimp should be opaque.
9. Remove the shrimp from the oven and serve with reserve sauce mixture and squeeze the lime wedges over.

470.Southwest Corn And Bell Pepper Roast

Servings: 4
Cooking Time: 10 Minutes
Ingredients:
- Corn:
- 1½ cups thawed frozen corn kernels
- 1 cup mixed diced bell peppers
- 1 jalapeño, diced
- 1 cup diced yellow onion
- ½ teaspoon ancho chile powder
- 1 tablespoon fresh lemon juice
- 1 teaspoon ground cumin
- ½ teaspoon kosher salt
- Cooking spray
- For Serving:
- ¼ cup feta cheese
- ¼ cup chopped fresh cilantro
- 1 tablespoon fresh lemon juice

Directions:
1. Spritz the air fryer basket with cooking spray.
2. Combine the ingredients for the corn in a large bowl. Stir to mix well.
3. Pour the mixture into the basket.
4. Put the air fryer basket on the baking pan and slide into Rack Position 2, select Air Fry, set temperature to 375ºF (190ºC) and set time to 10 minutes.
5. Stir the mixture halfway through the cooking time.
6. When done, the corn and bell peppers should be soft.
7. Transfer them onto a large plate, then spread with feta cheese and cilantro. Drizzle with lemon juice and serve.

471.Broccoli, Carrot, And Tomato Quiche

Servings: 4
Cooking Time: 14 Minutes
Ingredients:
- 4 eggs
- 1 teaspoon dried thyme
- 1 cup whole milk
- 1 steamed carrots, diced
- 2 cups steamed broccoli florets
- 2 medium tomatoes, diced
- ¼ cup crumbled feta cheese
- 1 cup grated Cheddar cheese
- 1 teaspoon chopped parsley
- Salt and ground black pepper, to taste
- Cooking spray

Directions:
1. Spritz the baking pan with cooking spray.
2. Whisk together the eggs, thyme, salt, and ground black pepper in a bowl and fold in the milk while mixing.
3. Put the carrots, broccoli, and tomatoes in the prepared baking pan, then spread with feta cheese and ½ cup Cheddar cheese. Pour the egg mixture over, then scatter with remaining Cheddar on top.
4. Slide the baking pan into Rack Position 1, select Convection Bake, set temperature to 350ºF (180ºC) and set time to 14 minutes.
5. When cooking is complete, the egg should be set and the quiche should be puffed.
6. Remove the quiche from the oven and top with chopped parsley, then slice to serve.

472.Traditional Latkes

Servings: 4 Latkes
Cooking Time: 10 Minutes
Ingredients:
- 1 egg
- 2 tablespoons all-purpose flour
- 2 medium potatoes, peeled and shredded, rinsed and drained
- ¼ teaspoon granulated garlic
- ½ teaspoon salt
- Cooking spray

Directions:
1. Spritz the air fryer basket with cooking spray.
2. Whisk together the egg, flour, potatoes, garlic, and salt in a large bowl. Stir to mix well.
3. Divide the mixture into four parts, then flatten them into four circles. Arrange the circles onto the basket and spritz with cooking spray.
4. Put the air fryer basket on the baking pan and slide into Rack Position 2, select Air Fry, set temperature to 380ºF (193ºC) and set time to 10 minutes.
5. Flip the latkes halfway through.
6. When cooked, the latkes will be golden brown and crispy. Remove from the oven and serve immediately.

473.Oven Grits

Servings: About 4 Cups
Cooking Time: 1 Hour 5 Minutes
Ingredients:
- 1 cup grits or polenta (not instant or quick cook)
- 2 cups chicken or vegetable stock
- 2 cups milk
- 2 tablespoons unsalted butter, cut into 4 pieces
- 1 teaspoon kosher salt or ½ teaspoon fine salt

Directions:

1. Add the grits to the baking pan. Stir in the stock, milk, butter, and salt.
2. Select Bake, set the temperature to 325ºF (163ºC), and set the time for 1 hour and 5 minutes. Select Start to begin preheating.
3. Once the unit has preheated, place the pan in the oven.
4. After 15 minutes, remove the pan from the oven and stir the polenta. Return the pan to the oven and continue cooking.
5. After 30 minutes, remove the pan again and stir the polenta again. Return the pan to the oven and continue cooking for 15 to 20 minutes, or until the polenta is soft and creamy and the liquid is absorbed.
6. When done, remove the pan from the oven.
7. Serve immediately.

474.Pastrami Casserole

Servings: 2
Cooking Time: 8 Minutes
Ingredients:
- 1 cup pastrami, sliced
- 1 bell pepper, chopped
- ¼ cup Greek yogurt
- 2 spring onions, chopped
- ½ cup Cheddar cheese, grated
- 4 eggs
- ¼ teaspoon ground black pepper
- Sea salt, to taste
- Cooking spray

Directions:
1. Spritz the baking pan with cooking spray.
2. Whisk together all the ingredients in a large bowl. Stir to mix well. Pour the mixture into the baking pan.
3. Slide the baking pan into Rack Position 1, select Convection Bake, set temperature to 330ºF (166ºC) and set time to 8 minutes.
4. When cooking is complete, the eggs should be set and the casserole edges should be lightly browned.
5. Remove from the oven and allow to cool for 10 minutes before serving.

475.Sweet And Sour Peanuts

Servings: 9
Cooking Time: 5 Minutes
Ingredients:
- 3 cups shelled raw peanuts
- 1 tablespoon hot red pepper sauce
- 3 tablespoons granulated white sugar

Directions:

1. Put the peanuts in a large bowl, then drizzle with hot red pepper sauce and sprinkle with sugar. Toss to coat well.
2. Pour the peanuts in the air fryer basket.
3. Put the air fryer basket on the baking pan and slide into Rack Position 2, select Air Fry, set temperature to 400ºF (205ºC) and set time to 5 minutes.
4. Stir the peanuts halfway through the cooking time.
5. When cooking is complete, the peanuts will be crispy and browned. Remove from the oven and serve immediately.

476.Riced Cauliflower Casserole

Servings: 4
Cooking Time: 12 Minutes
Ingredients:
- 1 head cauliflower, cut into florets
- 1 cup okra, chopped
- 1 yellow bell pepper, chopped
- 2 eggs, beaten
- ½ cup chopped onion
- 1 tablespoon soy sauce
- 2 tablespoons olive oil
- Salt and ground black pepper,
- to taste Spritz the baking pan with cooking spray.

Directions:
1. Put the cauliflower in a food processor and pulse to rice the cauliflower.
2. Pour the cauliflower rice in the baking pan and add the remaining ingredients. Stir to mix well.
3. Slide the baking pan into Rack Position 1, select Convection Bake, set temperature to 380ºF (193ºC) and set time to 12 minutes.
4. When cooking is complete, the eggs should be set.
5. Remove from the oven and serve immediately.

477.Classic Marinara Sauce

Servings: About 3 Cups
Cooking Time: 30 Minutes
Ingredients:
- ¼ cup extra-virgin olive oil
- 3 garlic cloves, minced
- 1 small onion, chopped (about ½ cup)
- 2 tablespoons minced or puréed sun-dried tomatoes (optional)
- 1 (28-ounce / 794-g) can crushed tomatoes
- ½ teaspoon dried basil
- ½ teaspoon dried oregano
- ¼ teaspoon red pepper flakes

Directions:

1. 1 teaspoon kosher salt or ½ teaspoon fine salt, plus more as needed
2. Heat the oil in a medium saucepan over medium heat.
3. Add the garlic and onion and sauté for 2 to 3 minutes, or until the onion is softened. Add the sun-dried tomatoes (if desired) and cook for 1 minute until fragrant. Stir in the crushed tomatoes, scraping any brown bits from the bottom of the pot. Fold in the basil, oregano, red pepper flakes, and salt. Stir well.
4. Bring to a simmer. Cook covered for about 30 minutes, stirring occasionally.
5. Turn off the heat and allow the sauce to cool for about 10 minutes.
6. Taste and adjust the seasoning, adding more salt if needed.
7. Use immediately.

478.Simple Butter Cake

Servings: 8
Cooking Time: 20 Minutes
Ingredients:
- 1 cup all-purpose flour
- 1¼ teaspoons baking powder
- ¼ teaspoon salt
- ½ cup plus 1½ tablespoons granulated white sugar
- 9½ tablespoons butter, at room temperature
- 2 large eggs
- 1 large egg yolk
- 2½ tablespoons milk
- 1 teaspoon vanilla extract
- Cooking spray

Directions:
1. Spritz the baking pan with cooking spray.
2. Combine the flour, baking powder, and salt in a large bowl. Stir to mix well.
3. Whip the sugar and butter in a separate bowl with a hand mixer on medium speed for 3 minutes.
4. Whip the eggs, egg yolk, milk, and vanilla extract into the sugar and butter mix with a hand mixer.
5. Pour in the flour mixture and whip with hand mixer until sanity and smooth.
6. Scrape the batter into the baking pan and level the batter with a spatula.
7. Slide the baking pan into Rack Position 1, select Convection Bake, set temperature to 325ºF (163ºC) and set time to 20 minutes.
8. After 15 minutes, remove the pan from the oven. Check the doneness. Return the pan to the oven and continue cooking.
9. When done, a toothpick inserted in the center should come out clean.

10. Invert the cake on a cooling rack and allow to cool for 15 minutes before slicing to serve.

479.Pão De Queijo

Servings: 12 Balls
Cooking Time: 12 Minutes
Ingredients:
- 2 tablespoons butter, plus more for greasing
- ½ cup milk
- 1½ cups tapioca flour
- ½ teaspoon salt
- 1 large egg
- $^2/_3$ cup finely grated aged Asiago cheese

Directions:
1. Put the butter in a saucepan and pour in the milk, heat over medium heat until the liquid boils. Keep stirring.
2. Turn off the heat and mix in the tapioca flour and salt to form a soft dough. Transfer the dough in a large bowl, then wrap the bowl in plastic and let sit for 15 minutes.
3. Break the egg in the bowl of dough and whisk with a hand mixer for 2 minutes or until a sanity dough forms. Fold the cheese in the dough. Cover the bowl in plastic again and let sit for 10 more minutes.
4. Grease the baking pan with butter.
5. Scoop 2 tablespoons of the dough into the baking pan. Repeat with the remaining dough to make dough 12 balls. Keep a little distance between each two balls.
6. Slide the baking pan into Rack Position 1, select Convection Bake, set temperature to 375ºF (190ºC) and set time to 12 minutes.
7. Flip the balls halfway through the cooking time.
8. When cooking is complete, the balls should be golden brown and fluffy.
9. Remove the balls from the oven and allow to cool for 5 minutes before serving.

480.Citrus Avocado Wedge Fries

Servings: 12 Fries
Cooking Time: 8 Minutes
Ingredients:
- 1 cup all-purpose flour
- 3 tablespoons lime juice
- ¾ cup orange juice
- 1¼ cups plain dried bread crumbs
- 1 cup yellow cornmeal
- 1½ tablespoons chile powder
- 2 large Hass avocados, peeled, pitted, and cut into wedges
- Coarse sea salt, to taste
- Cooking spray

Directions:
1. Spritz the air fryer basket with cooking spray.
2. Pour the flour in a bowl. Mix the lime juice with orange juice in a second bowl. Combine the bread crumbs, cornmeal, and chile powder in a third bowl.
3. Dip the avocado wedges in the bowl of flour to coat well, then dredge the wedges into the bowl of juice mixture, and then dunk the wedges in the bread crumbs mixture. Shake the excess off.
4. Arrange the coated avocado wedges in a single layer in the basket. Spritz with cooking spray.
5. Put the air fryer basket on the baking pan and slide into Rack Position 2, select Air Fry, set temperature to 400ºF (205ºC) and set time to 8 minutes.
6. Stir the avocado wedges and sprinkle with salt halfway through the cooking time.
7. When cooking is complete, the avocado wedges should be tender and crispy.
8. Serve immediately.

481.Classic Worcestershire Poutine

Servings: 2
Cooking Time: 33 Minutes
Ingredients:
- 2 russet potatoes, scrubbed and cut into ½-inch sticks
- 2 teaspoons vegetable oil
- 2 tablespoons butter
- ¼ onion, minced
- ¼ teaspoon dried thyme
- 1 clove garlic, smashed
- 3 tablespoons all-purpose flour
- 1 teaspoon tomato paste
- 1½ cups beef stock
- 2 teaspoons Worcestershire sauce
- Salt and freshly ground black pepper, to taste
- $^2/_3$ cup chopped string cheese

Directions:
1. Bring a pot of water to a boil, then put in the potato sticks and blanch for 4 minutes.
2. Drain the potato sticks and rinse under running cold water, then pat dry with paper towels.
3. Transfer the sticks in a large bowl and drizzle with vegetable oil. Toss to coat well. Place the potato sticks in the air fryer basket.
4. Put the air fryer basket on the baking pan and slide into Rack Position 2, select Air Fry, set temperature to 400ºF (205ºC) and set time to 25 minutes.
5. Stir the potato sticks at least three times during cooking.
6. Meanwhile, make the gravy: Heat the butter in a saucepan over medium heat until melted.

7. Add the onion, thyme, and garlic and sauté for 5 minutes or until the onion is translucent.
8. Add the flour and sauté for an additional 2 minutes. Pour in the tomato paste and beef stock and cook for 1 more minute or until lightly thickened.
9. Drizzle the gravy with Worcestershire sauce and sprinkle with salt and ground black pepper. Reduce the heat to low to keep the gravy warm until ready to serve.
10. When done, the sticks should be golden brown. Remove from the oven. Transfer the fried potato sticks onto a plate, then sprinkle with salt and ground black pepper. Scatter with string cheese and pour the gravy over. Serve warm.

482.Dehydrated Honey-rosemary Roasted Almonds

Ingredients:
- 1 heaping tablespoon demerara sugar
- 1 teaspoon finely chopped fresh rosemary
- 1 teaspoon kosher salt
- 8 ounces (225g) raw almonds
- 2 tablespoons kosher salt
- Honey-Rosemary glaze
- ¼ cup (80g) honey

Directions:
1. Place almonds and salt in a bowl. Add cold tap water to cover the almonds by 1-inch
2. (2cm). Let soak at room temperature for 12 hours to activate.
3. Rinse almonds under cold running water, then drain. Spread in a single layer on the dehydrate basket.
4. Dehydrate almonds for 24 hours or till tender and somewhat crispy but additionally spongy in the middle. Almonds may be eaten plain or roasted each the next recipe.
5. Put honey in a small saucepan and heat over Low heat. Put triggered nuts
6. At a medium bowl and then pour over warm honey. Stir To coat nuts equally. Add rosemary, sugar
7. And salt and stir to blend.
8. Spread Almonds in one layer on the skillet.
9. Insert cable rack into rack place 6. Select BAKE/350°F (175°C)/CONVECTION/10 moments and empower Rotate Remind.
10. Stirring almonds when Rotate Remind signs.
11. Let cool completely before storing in an airtight container.

483.Simple Air Fried Okra Chips

Servings: 6
Cooking Time: 16 Minutes

Ingredients:
- 2 pounds (907 g) fresh okra pods, cut into 1-inch pieces
- 2 tablespoons canola oil
- 1 teaspoon coarse sea salt

Directions:
1. Stir the oil and salt in a bowl to mix well. Add the okra and toss to coat well. Place the okra in the air fryer basket.
2. Put the air fryer basket on the baking pan and slide into Rack Position 2, select Air Fry, set temperature to 400ºF (205ºC) and set time to 16 minutes.
3. Flip the okra at least three times during cooking.
4. When cooked, the okra should be lightly browned. Remove from the oven and serve immediately.

484.Chicken Sausage And Broccoli Casserole

Servings: 8
Cooking Time: 20 Minutes
Ingredients:
- 10 eggs
- 1 cup Cheddar cheese, shredded and divided
- ¾ cup heavy whipping cream
- 1 (12-ounce / 340-g) package cooked chicken sausage
- 1 cup broccoli, chopped
- 2 cloves garlic, minced
- ½ tablespoon salt
- ¼ tablespoon ground black pepper
- Cooking spray

Directions:
1. Spritz the baking pan with cooking spray.
2. Whisk the eggs with Cheddar and cream in a large bowl to mix well.
3. Combine the cooked sausage, broccoli, garlic, salt, and ground black pepper in a separate bowl. Stir to mix well.
4. Pour the sausage mixture into the baking pan, then spread the egg mixture over to cover.
5. Slide the baking pan into Rack Position 1, select Convection Bake, set temperature to 400ºF (205ºC) and set time to 20 minutes.
6. When cooking is complete, the egg should be set and a toothpick inserted in the center should come out clean.
7. Serve immediately.

485.Air Fried Blistered Tomatoes

Servings: 4 To 6
Cooking Time: 10 Minutes

Ingredients:
- 2 pounds (907 g) cherry tomatoes
- 2 tablespoons olive oil
- 2 teaspoons balsamic vinegar
- ½ teaspoon salt
- ½ teaspoon ground black pepper

Directions:
1. Toss the cherry tomatoes with olive oil in a large bowl to coat well. Pour the tomatoes in the baking pan.
2. Put the air fryer basket on the baking pan and slide into Rack Position 2, select Air Fry, set temperature to 400ºF (205ºC) and set time to 10 minutes.
3. Stir the tomatoes halfway through the cooking time.
4. When cooking is complete, the tomatoes will be blistered and lightly wilted.
5. Transfer the blistered tomatoes to a large bowl and toss with balsamic vinegar, salt, and black pepper before serving.

486.Golden Salmon And Carrot Croquettes

Servings: 6
Cooking Time: 10 Minutes
Ingredients:
- 2 egg whites
- 1 cup almond flour
- 1 cup panko bread crumbs
- 1 pound (454 g) chopped salmon fillet
- $^2/_3$ cup grated carrots
- 2 tablespoons minced garlic cloves
- ½ cup chopped onion
- 2 tablespoons chopped chives
- Cooking spray

Directions:
1. Spritz the air fryer basket with cooking spray.
2. Whisk the egg whites in a bowl. Put the flour in a second bowl. Pour the bread crumbs in a third bowl. Set aside.
3. Combine the salmon, carrots, garlic, onion, and chives in a large bowl. Stir to mix well.
4. Form the mixture into balls with your hands. Dredge the balls into the flour, then egg, and then bread crumbs to coat well.
5. Arrange the salmon balls on the basket and spritz with cooking spray.
6. Put the air fryer basket on the baking pan and slide into Rack Position 2, select Air Fry, set temperature to 350ºF (180ºC) and set time to 10 minutes.
7. Flip the salmon balls halfway through cooking.
8. When cooking is complete, the salmon balls will be crispy and browned. Remove from the oven and serve immediately.

487.Crunchy And Beery Onion Rings

Servings: 2 To 4
Cooking Time: 16 Minutes
Ingredients:
- $^2/_3$ cup all-purpose flour
- 1 teaspoon paprika
- ½ teaspoon baking soda
- 1 teaspoon salt
- ½ teaspoon freshly ground black pepper
- 1 egg, beaten
- ¾ cup beer
- 1½ cups bread crumbs
- 1 tablespoons olive oil
- 1 large Vidalia onion, peeled and sliced into ½-inch rings
- Cooking spray

Directions:
1. Spritz the air fryer basket with cooking spray.
2. Combine the flour, paprika, baking soda, salt, and ground black pepper in a bowl. Stir to mix well.
3. Combine the egg and beer in a separate bowl. Stir to mix well.
4. Make a well in the center of the flour mixture, then pour the egg mixture in the well. Stir to mix everything well.
5. Pour the bread crumbs and olive oil in a shallow plate. Stir to mix well.
6. Dredge the onion rings gently into the flour and egg mixture, then shake the excess off and put into the plate of bread crumbs. Flip to coat the both sides well. Arrange the onion rings in the basket.
7. Put the air fryer basket on the baking pan and slide into Rack Position 2, select Air Fry, set temperature to 360ºF (182ºC) and set time to 16 minutes.
8. Flip the rings and put the bottom rings to the top halfway through.
9. When cooked, the rings will be golden brown and crunchy. Remove from the oven and serve immediately.

488.Classic Churros

Servings: 12 Churros
Cooking Time: 10 Minutes
Ingredients:
- 4 tablespoons butter
- ¼ teaspoon salt
- ½ cup water
- ½ cup all-purpose flour
- 2 large eggs
- 2 teaspoons ground cinnamon
- ¼ cup granulated white sugar
- Cooking spray

Directions:
1. Put the butter, salt, and water in a saucepan. Bring to a boil until the butter is melted on high heat. Keep stirring.
2. Reduce the heat to medium and fold in the flour to form a dough. Keep cooking and stirring until the dough is dried out and coat the pan with a crust.
3. Turn off the heat and scrape the dough in a large bowl. Allow to cool for 15 minutes.
4. Break and whisk the eggs into the dough with a hand mixer until the dough is sanity and firm enough to shape.
5. Scoop up 1 tablespoon of the dough and roll it into a ½-inch-diameter and 2-inch-long cylinder. Repeat with remaining dough to make 12 cylinders in total.
6. Combine the cinnamon and sugar in a large bowl and dunk the cylinders into the cinnamon mix to coat.
7. Arrange the cylinders on a plate and refrigerate for 20 minutes.
8. Spritz the air fryer basket with cooking spray. Place the cylinders in the basket and spritz with cooking spray.
9. Put the air fryer basket on the baking pan and slide into Rack Position 2, select Air Fry, set temperature to 375ºF (190ºC) and set time to 10 minutes.
10. Flip the cylinders halfway through the cooking time.
11. When cooked, the cylinders should be golden brown and fluffy.
12. Serve immediately.

489.Smoked Trout And Crème Fraiche Frittata

Servings: 4
Cooking Time: 17 Minutes
Ingredients:
- 2 tablespoons olive oil
- 1 onion, sliced
- 1 egg, beaten
- ½ tablespoon horseradish sauce
- 6 tablespoons crème fraiche
- 1 cup diced smoked trout
- 2 tablespoons chopped fresh dill
- Cooking spray

Directions:
1. Spritz the baking pan with cooking spray.
2. Heat the olive oil in a nonstick skillet over medium heat until shimmering.
3. Add the onion and sauté for 3 minutes or until translucent.

4. Combine the egg, horseradish sauce, and crème fraiche in a large bowl. Stir to mix well, then mix in the sautéed onion, smoked trout, and dill.
5. Pour the mixture in the prepared baking pan.
6. Slide the baking pan into Rack Position 1, select Convection Bake, set temperature to 350ºF (180ºC) and set time to 14 minutes.
7. Stir the mixture halfway through.
8. When cooking is complete, the egg should be set and the edges should be lightly browned.
9. Serve immediately.

490.Sumptuous Vegetable Frittata

Servings: 2
Cooking Time: 20 Minutes
Ingredients:
- 4 eggs
- $1/3$ cup milk
- 2 teaspoons olive oil
- 1 large zucchini, sliced
- 2 asparagus, sliced thinly
- $1/3$ cup sliced mushrooms
- 1 cup baby spinach
- 1 small red onion, sliced
- $1/3$ cup crumbled feta cheese
- $1/3$ cup grated Cheddar cheese
- ¼ cup chopped chives
- Salt and ground black pepper, to taste

Directions:
1. Line the baking pan with parchment paper.
2. Whisk together the eggs, milk, salt, and ground black pepper in a large bowl. Set aside.
3. Heat the olive oil in a nonstick skillet over medium heat until shimmering.
4. Add the zucchini, asparagus, mushrooms, spinach, and onion to the skillet and sauté for 5 minutes or until tender.
5. Pour the sautéed vegetables into the prepared baking pan, then spread the egg mixture over and scatter with cheeses.
6. Slide the baking pan into Rack Position 1, select Convection Bake, set temperature to 380ºF (193ºC) and set time to 15 minutes.
7. Stir the mixture halfway through.
8. When cooking is complete, the egg should be set and the edges should be lightly browned.
9. Remove the frittata from the oven and sprinkle with chives before serving.

491.Golden Nuggets

Servings: 20 Nuggets
Cooking Time: 4 Minutes
Ingredients:
- 1 cup all-purpose flour, plus more for dusting
- 1 teaspoon baking powder
- ½ teaspoon butter, at room temperature, plus more for brushing
- ¼ teaspoon salt
- ¼ cup water
- ⅛ teaspoon onion powder
- ¼ teaspoon garlic powder
- ⅛ teaspoon seasoning salt
- Cooking spray

Directions:
1. Line the air fryer basket with parchment paper.
2. Mix the flour, baking powder, butter, and salt in a large bowl. Stir to mix well. Gradually whisk in the water until a sanity dough forms.
3. Put the dough on a lightly floured work surface, then roll it out into a ½-inch thick rectangle with a rolling pin.
4. Cut the dough into about twenty 1- or 2-inch squares, then arrange the squares in a single layer in the basket. Spritz with cooking spray.
5. Combine onion powder, garlic powder, and seasoning salt in a small bowl. Stir to mix well, then sprinkle the squares with the powder mixture.
6. Put the air fryer basket on the baking pan and slide into Rack Position 2, select Air Fry, set temperature to 370ºF (188ºC) and set time to 4 minutes.
7. Flip the squares halfway through the cooking time.
8. When cooked, the dough squares should be golden brown.
9. Remove the golden nuggets from the oven and brush with more butter immediately. Serve warm.

492.Easy Corn And Bell Pepper Casserole

Servings: 4
Cooking Time: 20 Minutes
Ingredients:
- 1 cup corn kernels
- ¼ cup bell pepper, finely chopped
- ½ cup low-fat milk
- 1 large egg, beaten
- ½ cup yellow cornmeal
- ½ cup all-purpose flour
- ½ teaspoon baking powder
- 2 tablespoons melted unsalted butter
- 1 tablespoon granulated sugar
- Pinch of cayenne pepper
- ¼ teaspoon kosher salt
- Cooking spray

Directions:
1. Spritz the baking pan with cooking spray.

2. Combine all the ingredients in a large bowl. Stir to mix well. Pour the mixture into the baking pan.
3. Slide the baking pan into Rack Position 1, select Convection Bake, set temperature to 330ºF (166ºC) and set time to 20 minutes.
4. When cooking is complete, the casserole should be lightly browned and set.
5. Remove from the oven and serve immediately.

493.Teriyaki Shrimp Skewers

Servings: 12 Skewered Shrimp
Cooking Time: 6 Minutes
Ingredients:
- 1½ tablespoons mirin
- 1½ teaspoons ginger juice
- 1½ tablespoons soy sauce
- 12 large shrimp (about 20 shrimps per pound), peeled and deveined
- 1 large egg
- ¾ cup panko bread crumbs
- Cooking spray

Directions:
1. Combine the mirin, ginger juice, and soy sauce in a large bowl. Stir to mix well.
2. Dunk the shrimp in the bowl of mirin mixture, then wrap the bowl in plastic and refrigerate for 1 hour to marinate.
3. Spritz the air fryer basket with cooking spray.
4. Run twelve 4-inch skewers through each shrimp.
5. Whisk the egg in the bowl of marinade to combine well. Pour the bread crumbs on a plate.
6. Dredge the shrimp skewers in the egg mixture, then shake the excess off and roll over the bread crumbs to coat well.
7. Arrange the shrimp skewers in the basket and spritz with cooking spray.
8. Put the air fryer basket on the baking pan and slide into Rack Position 2, select Air Fry, set temperature to 400ºF (205ºC) and set time to 6 minutes.
9. Flip the shrimp skewers halfway through the cooking time.
10. When done, the shrimp will be opaque and firm.
11. Serve immediately.

494.Kale Frittata

Servings: 2
Cooking Time: 11 Minutes
Ingredients:
- 1 cup kale, chopped
- 1 teaspoon olive oil
- 4 large eggs, beaten
- Kosher salt, to taste
- 2 tablespoons water
- 3 tablespoons crumbled feta
- Cooking spray

Directions:
1. Spritz the baking pan with cooking spray.
2. Add the kale to the baking pan and drizzle with olive oil.
3. Slide the baking pan into Rack Position 2, select Convection Broil, set temperature to 360ºF (182ºC) and set time to 3 minutes.
4. Stir the kale halfway through.
5. When cooking is complete, the kale should be wilted.
6. Meanwhile, combine the eggs with salt and water in a large bowl. Stir to mix well.
7. Make the frittata: When broiling is complete, pour the eggs into the baking pan and spread with feta cheese.
8. Slide the baking pan into Rack Position 1, select Convection Bake, set temperature to 300ºF (150ºC) and set time to 8 minutes.
9. When cooking is complete, the eggs should be set and the cheese should be melted.
10. Remove from the oven and serve the frittata immediately.

495.Simple Baked Green Beans

Servings: 2 Cups
Cooking Time: 10 Minutes
Ingredients:
- ½ teaspoon lemon pepper
- 2 teaspoons granulated garlic
- ½ teaspoon salt
- 1 tablespoon olive oil
- 2 cups fresh green beans, trimmed and snapped in half

Directions:
1. Combine the lemon pepper, garlic, salt, and olive oil in a bowl. Stir to mix well.
2. Add the green beans to the bowl of mixture and toss to coat well.
3. Arrange the green beans in the the baking pan.
4. Slide the baking pan into Rack Position 1, select Convection Bake, set temperature to 370ºF (188ºC) and set time to 10 minutes.
5. Stir the green beans halfway through the cooking time.
6. When cooking is complete, the green beans will be tender and crispy. Remove from the oven and serve immediately.

496.Crispy Cheese Wafer

Servings: 2
Cooking Time: 5 Minutes

Ingredients:
- 1 cup shredded aged Manchego cheese
- 1 teaspoon all-purpose flour
- ½ teaspoon cumin seeds
- ¼ teaspoon cracked black pepper

Directions:
1. Line the air fryer basket with parchment paper.
2. Combine the cheese and flour in a bowl. Stir to mix well. Spread the mixture in the pan into a 4-inch round.
3. Combine the cumin and black pepper in a small bowl. Stir to mix well. Sprinkle the cumin mixture over the cheese round.
4. Put the air fryer basket on the baking pan and slide into Rack Position 2, select Air Fry, set temperature to 375ºF (190ºC) and set time to 5 minutes.
5. When cooked, the cheese will be lightly browned and frothy.
6. Use tongs to transfer the cheese wafer onto a plate and slice to serve.

497.Spicy Air Fried Old Bay Shrimp

Servings: 2 Cups
Cooking Time: 10 Minutes
Ingredients:
- ½ teaspoon Old Bay Seasoning
- 1 teaspoon ground cayenne pepper
- ½ teaspoon paprika
- 1 tablespoon olive oil
- ⅛ teaspoon salt
- ½ pound (227 g) shrimps, peeled and deveined
- Juice of half a lemon

Directions:
1. Combine the Old Bay Seasoning, cayenne pepper, paprika, olive oil, and salt in a large bowl, then add the shrimps and toss to coat well.
2. Put the shrimps in the air fryer basket.
3. Put the air fryer basket on the baking pan and slide into Rack Position 2, select Air Fry, set temperature to 390ºF (199ºC) and set time to 10 minutes.
4. Flip the shrimps halfway through the cooking time.
5. When cooking is complete, the shrimps should be opaque. Serve the shrimps with lemon juice on top.

498.Butternut Squash With Hazelnuts

Servings: 3 Cups
Cooking Time: 23 Minutes
Ingredients:
- 2 tablespoons whole hazelnuts

- 3 cups butternut squash, peeled, deseeded and cubed
- ¼ teaspoon kosher salt
- ¼ teaspoon freshly ground black pepper
- 2 teaspoons olive oil
- Cooking spray

Directions:
1. Spritz the air fryer basket with cooking spray. Spread the hazelnuts in the pan.
2. Put the air fryer basket on the baking pan and slide into Rack Position 2, select Air Fry, set temperature to 300ºF (150ºC) and set time to 3 minutes.
3. When done, the hazelnuts should be soft. Remove from the oven. Chopped the hazelnuts roughly and transfer to a small bowl. Set aside.
4. Put the butternut squash in a large bowl, then sprinkle with salt and pepper and drizzle with olive oil. Toss to coat well. Transfer the squash to the lightly greased basket.
5. Put the air fryer basket on the baking pan and slide into Rack Position 2, select Air Fry, set temperature to 360ºF (182ºC) and set time to 20 minutes.
6. Flip the squash halfway through the cooking time.
7. When cooking is complete, the squash will be soft. Transfer the squash to a plate and sprinkle with the chopped hazelnuts before serving.

499.Buttery Knots With Parsley

Servings: 8 Knots
Cooking Time: 5 Minutes
Ingredients:
- 1 teaspoon dried parsley
- ¼ cup melted butter
- 2 teaspoons garlic powder

Directions:
1. 1 (11-ounce / 312-g) tube refrigerated French bread dough, cut into 8 slices
2. Combine the parsley, butter, and garlic powder in a bowl. Stir to mix well.
3. Place the French bread dough slices on a clean work surface, then roll each slice into a 6-inch long rope. Tie the ropes into knots and arrange them on a plate.
4. Transfer the knots into the baking pan. Brush the knots with butter mixture.
5. Put the air fryer basket on the baking pan and slide into Rack Position 2, select Air Fry, set temperature to 350ºF (180ºC) and set time to 5 minutes.
6. Flip the knots halfway through the cooking time.
7. When done, the knots should be golden brown. Remove from the oven and serve immediately.

500.Creamy Pork Gratin

Servings: 4
Cooking Time: 21 Minutes
Ingredients:
- 2 tablespoons olive oil
- 2 pounds (907 g) pork tenderloin, cut into serving-size pieces
- 1 teaspoon dried marjoram
- ¼ teaspoon chili powder
- 1 teaspoon coarse sea salt
- ½ teaspoon freshly ground black pepper
- 1 cup Ricotta cheese
- 1½ cups chicken broth
- 1 tablespoon mustard
- Cooking spray

Directions:

1. Spritz the baking pan with cooking spray.
2. Heat the olive oil in a nonstick skillet over medium-high heat until shimmering.
3. Add the pork and sauté for 6 minutes or until lightly browned.
4. Transfer the pork to the prepared baking pan and sprinkle with marjoram, chili powder, salt, and ground black pepper.
5. Combine the remaining ingredients in a large bowl. Stir to mix well. Pour the mixture over the pork in the pan.
6. Slide the baking pan into Rack Position 1, select Convection Bake, set temperature to 350ºF (180ºC) and set time to 15 minutes.
7. Stir the mixture halfway through.
8. When cooking is complete, the mixture should be frothy and the cheese should be melted.
9. Serve immediately.